15,00

GREEN FOR LIFE

GREEN
FOR
Life

VICTORIA
BOUTENKO, M.A.

FOREWORD BY
A. WILLIAM MENZIN, M.D.

www.NaturalZing.com
1-888-Raw-Zing (729-9464)
info@naturalzing.com

Raw Family Publishing

Dedication

I dedicate this book to Dr. Ann Wigmore and others
who dare to think for themselves.

Raw Family Publishing
www.rawfamily.com

Library of Congress Control Number: 2005906308

ISBN 978-0-9704819-6-2

Disclaimer: The information contained in this book is not intended as
medical advice. Victoria Boutenko does not recommend cooked foods
or standard medical practices. The authors, publishers and/or
distributors will not assume responsibility for any adverse consequences
resulting from adopting the lifestyle described herein.

This book has been translated into the following languages: Russian,
German, Portuguese, French, Chinese, and Hungarian.

Contents

Foreword

In more than thirty-five years of practice as a psychiatrist affiliated with the Harvard Medical School, I have learned one thing well: Human behavior is very hard to change.

Now Victoria Boutenko is persuading me otherwise. Because this remarkable woman has developed a strategy for helping ordinary Americans (the ones who love ice cream and steak and French fries and pizza) introduce green living foods into their life in a delicious and habit-forming way. Nothing she says in her book, *Green for Life* — about our bodies' ability to restore itself to good health if given the right nutrients to work with — is exactly new in itself. And yet *Green for Life* is a groundbreaking achievement because Mrs. Boutenko has understood that the way to encourage her readers to trigger their natural mechanisms for cleaning cholesterol, fat and toxins from their bodies — and thereby to improve first their physical, and then their mental and spiritual, lives — is not to lecture her readers about the need to consume more living plant life, but to make it easy and pleasant for them to do it.

The green smoothie — or, to be more specific, the quart of green smoothie with which Mrs. Boutenko recommends

in this book that we all start our day—is in and of itself a
tremendous injection of chlorophyll, vitamins, minerals,
enzymes and antioxidants into the typical American diet. A
quart of green smoothie a day also discourages consumption
of denatured and greasy foods. For one thing, it's hard to
stuff yourself with refined starches and sugars when you're
full of one of Mrs. Boutenko's tasty and energizing concoc-
tions. (Check out one of the seventeen tempting recipes for
Sweet Green Smoothies on page 159.) And if another seduc-
tive green smoothie is waiting for you in the refrigerator
when you get home from work, the dinner you prepare and
consume after sipping it will almost certainly be smaller, and
possibly healthier, too.

Thirty days of green smoothies will also change how you
feel, and how you feel about yourself. That's no small
achievement for one small book.

I salute Mrs. Boutenko. I recommend that you take *Green
for Life* very seriously.

I believe it can help you change your life.

A. William Menzin, M.D.
Department of Psychiatry
Harvard Medical School
Former consultant to the World Health Organization (WHO)

Author's Note

Dear Reader,

I am delighted to share this book with you. In the following chapters I disclose many astonishing facts about greens and explain why they are the most essential part of human nutrition. Ever since I realized the key to radiant health was under my very nose, I began to read every book on greens I could get my hands on.

Initially, I only wanted to improve the classic raw food diet. Surprisingly, in the process of my research, I found that adding blended greens to anyone's diet makes such a profound health improvement, that it may even surpass the benefits of eating a typical all-raw diet with a relatively small amount of greens. In addition, drinking smoothies is by far more doable than switching at once to an all-raw diet. At the same time, I have discovered that people who incorporate blended greens into their daily meals naturally begin to eat more live foods.

Blended green smoothies are a simple and delicious way of accessing the healing properties of greens. Whether you eat a raw food, vegan, vegetarian, or mainstream American diet, regularly drinking green smoothies can significantly improve your health. This miraculous drink is available to every person in every country. Join me in discovering why greens are the perfect human food. I hope this information is as refreshing for you as it has been for me.

Victoria Boutenko

Acknowledgments

To my beloved husband Igor, for always being extraordinarily dependable in all my endeavors, for listening and discussing countless new concepts with me, and for his endless passion for truth. To my daughter Valya, for her graceful patience and dedication in clarifying the wording of this book. To my son Sergei, for his enthusiastic support and eloquent critiques. To my son Stephan, for his valuable insights, and inspiring phone calls.

To Dr. Paul Fieber and his wife Susie for their active help in organizing and conducting the Roseburg study. To all the participants of the Roseburg study for their time and commitment. To Vanessa Nowitzky, for her quick fingers, impeccable grammar, and sweet sense of humor. To Laura Hamilton, Shawna Huggins, and Kendall Olson Cassidy for the long hours they spent editing this manuscript. To Elizabeth Bechtold, Phyllis Linn, Offek Ohn-bar, Graham W. Boyes, Penny Budinsky, Daniel and Judy Sapon-Borson for their generous financial support of my research and the publishing of this book. To all those who sent me their enthusiastic endorsements. Thank you. May you all benefit from drinking green smoothies.

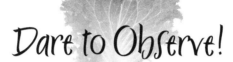

Dare to Observe!

"Doubt is the father of invention."
GALILEO GALILEI

Observation constitutes the foundation of every science. You and I, like everyone on this planet, have the right to make observations and draw our own conclusions whether we are scientists or not. Our personal experimentation helps us stay in charge of our own lives. No scientific data can substitute for our own experience.

When a child is told not to touch the fire, this warning doesn't mean much until he or she actually tries touching the flames and gets hurt. Only through observation can we learn to connect consequences with causes, to become aware of what to expect. For example, if we overeat late at night, we should not expect to feel fresh in the morning. The advantage of being aware of what is going to happen enables us to act deliberately in our everyday lives and **to achieve the goals we desire through conscious actions**, instead of constantly and blindly following the advice of somebody "who knows better."

I was raised in the Soviet Union where everyone was severely controlled by the government structures. Since early childhood, I was given firm instructions about what I was supposed to do, think, and even say. I was afraid to try anything new. However, I was very lucky to meet many incredible people in my life from whom I learned to dare to try everything I wanted.

I absolutely have to tell you about Alexander Suvorov whom I met several times and who became my hero and inspiration for many years. Alexander became totally blind and deaf when he was three years old. Nevertheless, he was so eager to live his life to the fullest that he learned to speak and to understand what other people were saying by holding their hands. He graduated from high school with an excellent diploma, then graduated as Ph.D. from Moscow University, wrote a number of brilliant scientific articles about helping blind and deaf children, published several books, and created a 40-minute documentary about his perception of life. This film gathered huge crowds in Moscow in the 70s. People were deeply impressed by Alexander's sincerity and passion. I remember that after the movie was over, nobody left the theater for a long time. We just sat there bewildered, sobbing, and ashamed of our cowardly lives and stupid fears. Alexander Suvorov, living his life in physical darkness and constant silence, had a dream to travel to other countries. So he learned two foreign languages and traveled to several countries on his own. When people asked him why he went, he replied that he wanted "to see the world for himself."

When I meet incredible human beings, like Alexander, or read about people who dare to "see for themselves," I begin to want to explore life around me more completely and to know how far my limits can stretch.

As we live our lives, trying new things and searching for true answers, we gain plenty of our own experiences. Our knowledge becomes familiar and practical. We feel rather confident in any life circumstance particularly when we need to make urgent decisions. Contrary to that, when all we have is a compilation of someone else's instructions, the best we can do is to hope and pray that the authors of such instructions were efficient in acquiring their knowledge and honest in their intentions. In other words **we hope that someone else cares for us more than we care for our own selves.**

When we let others observe and reason for us, in a sense, we consciously choose to stay blind and deaf. We become compelled to follow someone else's instructions, one after another, and perform actions which do not make much sense to us. We submit to other's authority. We give our power away.

To observe is our birthright. If we utilize our ability to observe, we can free ourselves from the labyrinth of confusions. I believe that our own conscious observations are a thousand times more important than any rigid scientific claim.

Why have so many books on nutrition been published lately? Obviously there is a big question from the public about health that has not been satisfied by the scientific wing of our world community. Most of us are totally cut off from researchers, and at the same time, scientists are disconnected from ordinary people. I wonder why this has happened, since the original goal of science is human well-being.

Most results of pure science are unavailable and unaffordable for common people. For example, in order to obtain a two or three page report from nearly all medical studies, I had to pay a lot of money, sometimes hundreds of dollars for each of them. The average research paper is written in complex, scientific terms, which makes it incomprehensible to people who don't belong to this particular branch of science. I have observed that the branches of science are increasing in number and the language they use continually multiplies in terms. Throughout my life I have spoken to dozens of different scientists in different parts of the world and I have never met one scientist who was able to understand and explain studies from all the branches at the same time. In fact, the more scientists claim to know about one subject the more they tend to say, "That's not my field" about the others.

This tendency suggests that science is moving beyond the understanding of the average human beings towards **science for the sake of science**. While the public wants to know the newest achievements, the scientific world becomes less and less available for their burning inquiries. The informational vacuum begins to grow, especially in the field of health and nutrition.

To substitute for this missing, yet so needed information, the public begins to make its own science. It may not be completely accurate, but it is understandable to the majority of people. Hence, we witness hundreds if not thousands of books on nutrition written by average people, who undertake different research studies, sometimes without the necessary background. Being desperate for answers to their questions, people absorb this abundance of information and often get more confused.

I notice that many people trust the written word more than the spoken word. Due to the lack of people's own observations and a tendency to take whole concepts as if they were set in stone, health seekers embrace a certain concept, often depending on which book they have read first. As multitudes of nutritional books are generated, they begin to contradict one another. As a result, it is possible to encounter hundreds of people today with completely different suggestions of what to eat, all with hundreds of different reasons that cancel out each other.

When I started to do research about greens, I instantly and hopelessly sank into an ocean of information. In my situation I had *to find the true answer or die*. I felt responsible not only for my husband and my children whom I dragged onto the raw food diet with me, but all those thousands of people in the world that I inspired to adopt an all-raw diet. Finally, I decided to put everything aside for several months, and to sit down and read through as many original research papers as I could get on the subject of nutrition. I decided to cut away all the opinions and focus only on the original data because human reasoning can build up logical chains of thought that smoothly direct the reader to totally incorrect conclusions with devastating results. (Later in my book I will give examples of such mistakes in which I myself got trapped.)

I discovered that there were some substantial gaps in data, and there were numerous important foods whose qualities have never been studied. I realized that if I wanted to draw the right conclusions I had to initiate at least some pilot studies by myself. After all, my life was already an experiment in which I was the guinea pig.

I strongly believe, now more than ever, that it is safer to go on raw food for two weeks and see for oneself how one feels, than to read ten books and follow their recommendations without having any idea why. Through our careful observations we all have the ability to clearly see the results of our actions.

Dear reader! With this book I hope to inspire you to start observing which of your actions make you feel and look the healthiest and as a result to create your own personal plan that will work for you in the best way. You are your own best expert.

CHAPTER TWO

What was Missing in Our Raw Food Plan?

My husband, our two youngest children, and I have been eating an only raw foods diet since January of 1994, more than eleven years. We went on this radical diet out of complete despair when our medical doctors didn't leave us any chances to recover from our horrible illnesses.

My husband, Igor, had been constantly ill since his early childhood. By the tender age of 17 he had already survived nine surgeries. Having progressive hyperthyroidism and chronic rheumatoid arthritis, at 38 he was a total health wreck. I had to lace his shoes on rainy days because his arthritic spine would not bend. Igor's heart rate was 140+ most of the time, his eyes were tearing on sunny days and his hands were shaky. Igor constantly felt fatigued and was in pain almost all the time. Igor's "thyroid" doctor told him that he would die in less than two months if he would not agree to have his thyroid gland removed. His "arthritis" doctor told him to prepare to spend the rest of his life in a wheel chair.

I was diagnosed with the same disease that took my father; arrhythmia, or an irregular heart beat. My legs were constantly swollen from edema, I weighed 280 pounds, and I was continuously gaining more. My left arm frequently became numb at night and I was afraid that I would die and my children would become orphans. I remember always feeling tired and depressed.

Our daughter Valya was born with asthma and allergies and would often cough heavily all through the night. Our son Sergei was diagnosed with juvenile type 1 diabetes.

One day, after crying through the entire night, I decided that we had to take a *different* action if we wanted to get *different* results. That was when we started to try various healing modalities and eventually arrived at the idea of becoming raw foodists. At the time we didn't know anything about making fancy raw dishes or even that we could dehydrate flax crackers. Nevertheless, by turning off the pilot in our stove and discontinuing all cooking, we were able to heal all of our incurable, life-threatening diseases. Our health was improving so quickly that in three and a half months all four of us ran the Bolder Boulder 10K road race with the 40,000 other runners.

Even Sergei's blood sugar stabilized due to his new diet and regular jogging. Since beginning to eat raw food, he has never again experienced any form of diabetic symptoms. We were greatly surprised not only by how quickly our health was restored to normal, but by how much healthier we were than ever before. We have described the detailed story of our miraculous healing in our book *Raw Family: A True Story of Awakening*.

After several years of being raw foodists, however, each one of us began to feel like we had reached a plateau where our healing process stopped and even somewhat began to go backwards. After approximately seven years on a completely raw diet, once in a while, more and more often, we started feeling discontent with our existing food program. I began to have a heavy feeling in my stomach after eating almost any kind of raw food, especially a salad with dressing. Because of that, I started to eat less greens and more fruits and nuts. I began to gain weight. My husband started to develop a lot of gray hair. My family members felt confused about our diet and seemed often to have the question, "what should we eat?" There were odd times when we felt hungry but did not desire any foods that were "legal" for us to eat on a typical raw food diet: fruits, nuts, seeds, grains or dried fruit. Salads (with dressings) were delicious but made us tired and sleepy. We felt trapped. I remember Igor looking inside the fridge, saying over and over again, "I wish I wanted some of this stuff".... Such periods did not last. We blamed it all on overeating and were able to refresh our appetites by fasts, exercise, hikes or by working more. In my family we strongly believe that raw food is the *only way to go* and therefore we encouraged each other to maintain our raw diet no matter what, always coming up with new tricks. Many of my friends told me about similar experiences at which point they gave up being 100% raw and began to add cooked food back into their meals. In my family, we continued to stay on raw food due to our constant support of each other.

A burning question began to grow stronger in my heart with each day. The question was, "Is there anything missing in our diet?" The answer would come right away: "Nope. Nothing could be better than a raw food diet."

Yet, however tiny, the unwanted signs of less than perfect health kept surfacing in minor but noticeable symptoms such as a wart on a hand or a gray hair that brought doubts and questions about the completeness of the raw food diet in its present form. Finally, when my children complained about the increased sensitivity of their teeth, I reached a state where I couldn't think about anything besides this health puzzle. I drove everybody around me crazy with my constant discussion of what could possibly be missing.

In my eager quest, I started collecting data about every single food that existed for humans. As my grandmother used to say, "Seek and ye shall find." After many wrong guesses, I finally found the correct answer. I found one particular food group that matched ALL human nutritional needs: *greens*. The truth is, in my family, we were not eating enough greens. Moreover, we did not like them. We knew that greens were important, but we never heard anywhere exactly how much greens we needed in our diet. We had only a vague recommendation to eat as much as possible. In order to find out how much greens we needed to eat, I decided to study the eating habits of chimpanzees since they are one of the closest creatures to human beings.

CHAPTER THREE

How Chimpanzees Eat

C himpanzees are very similar to humans. Scientists at the Chimpanzee & Human Communication Institute at Washington Central University believe that "chimpanzees should be categorized as a people."[1] After closely studying the behavior of these intelligent beings, the researchers at WCU have become convinced that chimpanzees are significantly smarter than most people are aware. According to the scientists from WCU, chimpanzees have their own language and culture that humans didn't even suspect of them, probably because chimpanzees do not speak. They do, however, use their own sign language that scientists have been studying closely for over three decades. The researchers at WCU acknowledge: "New evidence indicates that the technology and the communication of the chimpanzee community meets the definition of culture. We also know that chimpanzee's cognitive capacities are very similar to our own,

both intellectually and emotionally. By any reasonable definition **chimpanzees should be categorized as a people**."[2]

Most medical research institutes agree that chimpanzees
and humans are very alike. Unfortunately, based on this
ground, they use chimpanzees in scientific experiments. Just
take a look at the following quotes from numerous medical
articles.

"Modern people and chimpanzees share an estimated
99.4% of our DNA sequence, making us more closely
related to each other than either is to any other animal
species."[3]

"Chimpanzees resemble humans more than any other
animal ... Human brains are very like chimpanzee brains.
The major differences between humans and apes are not
anatomical, but rather behavioral."[4]

"Chimps have the same A–B–O blood groupings as
humans and are used for compatibility studies for tissue
transplants, for hepatitis research and for other medical
studies."[5]

"Nonhuman primates [play a] critical role in biomedical
research of understanding, treatment and prevention of
important infectious diseases such as A.I.D.S., hepatitis, and
malaria, and chronic degenerative disorders of the central
nervous system (like Parkinson's and Alzheimer's diseases.)
... The close phylogenetic relation of NHPs to humans not
only opens avenues for testing the safety and efficacy of new
drugs and vaccines but also offers promise for evaluating the
potential of new gene-based treatments for human infectious
and genetic diseases."[6]

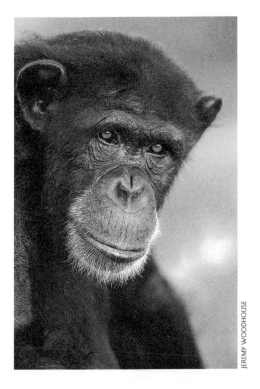

JEREMY WOODHOUSE

"Nonhuman primates are excellent models for studying human biology and behavior because of their close phylogenetic relation to humans. Their use in biomedical research is critical to advancements in medical science . . . [including] the discovery of the Rh factor and the development of the poliovirus vaccine . . . . Their use has expanded into virtually every area of medicine."[7]

I wonder, if chimpanzees and humans are really so closely related, and studying this closeness is so critical to our health, *why don't we humans apply our studies both ways?* How could it be that we put our worst human illnesses on chimpanzees but do not learn from them?

Rather than making them sick, why not make ourselves
well? Why not at least try out what they eat?

I went online and purchased $300 worth of books and
DVDs about chimpanzees and their diet and lifestyle. I wrote
a letter with my questions to the Jane Goodall University. I
traveled to three big zoos that have chimpanzees and spoke
to many people who feed them and take care of them every
day. I discovered fascinating information about chimpanzees
that totally changed my view of them.

I was very impressed to find out that chimpanzees can
learn to use American Sign Language:

"Under double-blind conditions, we have found that the
chimpanzees communicate information in American Sign
Language (ASL) to human observers. They use signs to refer
to natural language categories: e.g. DOG for any dog,
FLOWER for any flower, SHOE for any shoe, etc. The chimpanzees acquire and spontaneously use their signs to communicate with humans and each other about the normal
course of surrounding events. They have demonstrated an
ability to invent new signs or combine signs to metaphori-
cally label a novel item, for example: calling a radish CRY
HURT FOOD or referring to a watermelon as a DRINK
FRUIT. In a double-blind condition, the chimpanzees can
comprehend and produce novel prepositional phrases,
understand vocal English words, translate words into their
ASL glosses and even transmit their signing skills to the next
generation without human intervention. Their play behavior
has demonstrated that they use the same types of imaginary
play as humans. It has also been demonstrated that they

carry on chimpanzee-to-chimpanzee conversation and sign to themselves when alone. Conversational research shows the chimpanzees initiate and maintain conversations in ways that are like humans. The chimpanzees can repair a conversation if there is misunderstanding. They will also sign to themselves when alone and we have even observed them to sign in their sleep."[8]

When I educated myself about chimpanzees, they became one of my favorite beings. Understanding their intelligent nature, I feel deeply sorry for the 1,500 chimps that spend their lives in tiny indoor cages in medical laboratories in the United States.

Despite all the scientific research, human health is continuously declining. Many nutritionists connect human health problems with nutritional deficiencies. Humans have lost their natural way of eating. That is why I am so grateful that there is another species in this world that closely resembles us. In particular, I was glad to know that there are thousands of chimpanzees living in Gombe Valley, Africa. The most remarkable fact is that the majority of the chimps of Gombe, [as opposed to humans] have not been touched by civilization. That is a great fortune for us humans! It gives us hope to find the answers to our most vital questions: What is the human diet supposed to be? What was it originally?

Understanding chimpanzees' eating habits may help us better understand human dietary needs. Please look at this chart showing the average diet of the chimpanzee in the wilderness, that I created based on the data from Jane Goodall's book:

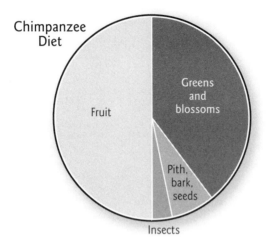

Chimpanzee Diet

As you can see, the two major food groups for chimpanzees are fruits and greens. Please do not confuse greens with root vegetables like carrots, beets, or potatoes. Also do not confuse greens with non-sweet fruits like cucumbers, tomatoes, zucchini, and bell peppers. Chimps only eat root vegetables in the case of drought or famine as a fall-back food.[9] According to Jane Goodall, a world famous researcher of chimpanzees, the percentage of time that chimpanzees spend eating greens in relation to the rest of their diet varies from 25–50% depending on the season.[10] Two to seven percent of their diet is pith and bark. (Piths are the stems and more fibrous parts of plants.) When the trees are blooming, in March and April, chimpanzees consume blossoms, up to 10% of their ratio. Chimpanzees do not eat very many nuts, but their diet could be up to 5% seeds. Also, particularly in November, they consume small amounts of insects and even small animals, however, Goodall says this part of their diet is irregular and insignificant, as they could go months and months without consuming any animals, and seem to have no ill effects. There is other research that points out that wild chimpanzees' intake of insects and other animals never comprises more than 1% of their diet.[11]

As long as I can remember, chimpanzees have been depicted with a banana or an orange in their hands, which definitely misled me to the assumption that they eat only fruit. To know that greens compose almost half of their diet was a revelation for me. My research gave me a solid idea that humans are supposed to eat far more greens than I would have guessed.

Let us compare the standard American diet with the diet of chimpanzees. As you can see they look totally different. These two diets hardly have anything in common! We humans eat mostly things that chimpanzees don't eat at all, like cooked starchy foods, oils, butter, yogurt, cheese, hamburgers, etc. While most of our vegetables are roots, wild chimpanzees almost never eat root vegetables unless there is a drought and fruits and greens are unavailable. It is the intake of greens that has declined most dramatically in the human diet. Our

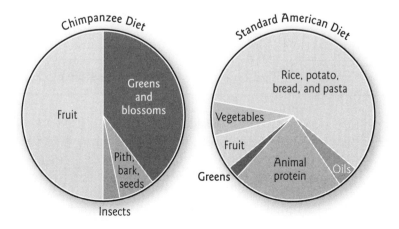

consumption of greens has generally shrunk to the two wilt-
ed iceberg lettuce leaves on our sandwich.

Let us compare the standard American diet with an average diet of a typical raw foodist.

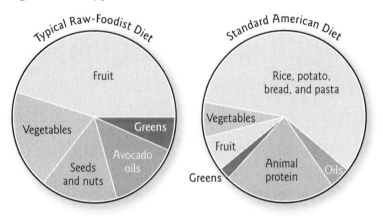

I think that a raw food diet demonstrates a vast improvement over the regular diet. Firstly, all ingredients in a raw
diet are uncooked, and full of enzymes and vitamins; thus
the raw food diet is like a revolution in comparison with the
standard American diet. That explains why so many people
reported that they instantly felt better on a raw diet. We can
see that raw fooders eat a lot of fruit, especially if we keep in
mind that bell-peppers, cucumbers, zucchini, and tomatoes
are also fruits. However, even though raw-foodists typically
consume noticeably more greens than people on an average
mainstream diet, greens almost never constitute 45 percent
of their food. So what do raw foodists eat in place of their
missing greens? The answer is: most people on a raw food
diet consume large amounts of fruits, nuts and seeds. Often
they use nuts as a substitute for carbohydrates, particularly
when trying to mimic cooked dishes with raw ingredients,

even though nuts are 70–80% fat. Also, raw foodists increase their consumption of oils and avocados because the most common way of eating salads, their main staple, is to have it mixed with dressing, sauce or guacamole. Another big quota in a typical raw diet belongs to root vegetables mostly due to juicing. Also, roots taste sweeter than greens and thus comprise a large portion of raw salads.

Considering all of these factors, when we compare the typical raw food diet with the chimpanzee diet, we can clearly see that there are two main ways to further improve our individual eating patterns: to increase our consumption of greens, and to reduce our intake of nuts, seeds, and oils.

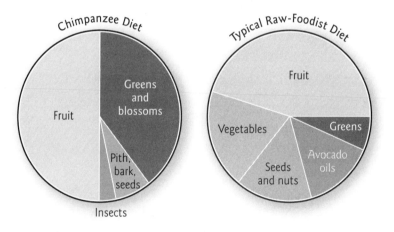

For example, based on how much fruit we consume in my family (about 4 or 5 pounds per day per person) I estimate that we need to eat about two good sized bunches of dark leafy greens per person per day.

Another striking characteristic aspect of the chimpanzee eating pattern is that they never eat in the late afternoon or evening. Chimpanzees wake up very early, at the first light of dawn. After leaving their nests, they groom each other for few minutes and then begin searching for food. Chimpanzees have to work hard in order to get their food, climbing many trees or searching through numerous low shrubs. Most often they feed on fruit in the morning and a little bit on leaves. After about four hours, they take a break for an hour or two, playing or sleeping in the sun. Then the chimps resume feeding, eating mostly greens until about three or four o'clock in the afternoon, after which they groom and prepare their nests for the night sleep.

In contrast, my own eating pattern is vastly different. I don't normally eat anything until noon or later, and in the evening I stock up on food. I am currently striving to stop eating after 6 p. m. While I am experiencing positive results and finally shedding some extra weight, I have to admit that restraining myself from eating late is a lot harder than I expected. I attribute this to the larger amount of stress we tend to accumulate towards the end of the day.

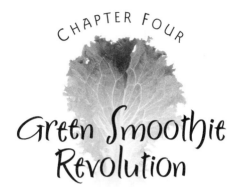

CHAPTER FOUR

Green Smoothie Revolution

*I*n my research, I noticed that chimpanzees really *love* greens. I remember watching chimps at the zoo and seeing how excited they became when given fresh acacia branches, young tender palm tree leaves, or kale. I was so inspired looking at them that I went to the nearby bushes and tried to eat acacia leaves myself. But the truth was, the green leaves were not very palatable for me and that presented another problem. Eating greens always seemed like a duty for me. I would think to myself, "I have to have my greens." Some days I would "cheat" by juicing my greens. I would quickly drink a cup of green juice and consider myself good for a couple of days. Or I would make a delicious raw dressing and sink my greens into it. That was another way for me to enjoy greens. But I could never imagine sitting and eating two bunches of kale or spinach.

Although I didn't like greens, my husband, Igor, simply couldn't tolerate them. When he was growing up he was encouraged to eat mostly meat and bread, "like a real Russian man." While living in Russia we had never seen any greens in stores. Only in the summer people could buy dill, parsley, and green onions at farmers markets. I recall seeing lettuce only about twice each summer and considered it rare and exotic.

The more I read about the nutritional content of greens, the more I became convinced that greens were the most important food for humans. If I could only find a way to enjoy them enough to consume the optimal quantity needed to become perfectly healthy!

I tried countless times to force myself to eat large amounts of greens in the form of salad or by themselves, only to discover that I was not physically able to do that. After about two cups of shredded greens I would either have heartburn or nausea.

One day, while reading a book on biology, I became intrigued by the amazingly hardy composition of plants. Apparently, cellulose, the main constituent of plants, has one of the strongest molecular structures on the planet. Greens possess more valuable nutrients than any other food group, but all these nutrients are stored inside the cells of plants. These cells are made of tough material, probably as a means of survival for the plant, making it difficult for animals to eat. **To release all the valuable nutrients from within the the cells, the cell walls need to be ruptured.** To rupture these sturdy cells is not easy. This is why eating greens without chewing them thoroughly would not satisfy our nutritional needs. In simple words, we need to chew our greens to a creamy consistency in order to get the benefits.

In addition, in order to digest the released minerals and vitamins, hydrochloric acid in the stomach has to be very strong, with a pH between 1 and 2.

These two conditions are absolutely, vitally, necessary for the assimilation of nutrients from greens. Obviously, when I tried to eat plain greens I did not chew my greens well enough and possibly did not have a high enough level of hydrochloric acid in my stomach. As a result, I experienced unpleasant signs of indigestion and formed a general dislike for greens altogether.

After many decades of eating mostly heavily processed foods, modern people have lost their ability to chew normally.[12] Our jaws have become so narrow that even after extracting our wisdom teeth, we still need to wear braces.[13] Our jaw muscles have become too weak to thoroughly chew rough fiber. Several times I have heard recommendations from my dentist to be more gentle on my teeth, and not to bite firm fruit, but rather to grate my carrots and apples. In addition to these compromising conditions, many people have lots of fillings, false, or missing teeth. All of these obstacles make chewing greens to the necessary consistency virtually impossible.

This is why I decided to try to "chew" my greens in the Vitamix blender.* First I blended a bunch of kale with

---

* I would like to explain that the Vitamix as well as the Blendtec are not like the blenders you can find at any department store. They are called high speed blenders, because their speed goes up to 240 mph! That means that their blades don't even have to be sharp; even if they were just dull metal sticks they could still liquefy something as hard as, for example, blocks of wood. In order to reach such performance, both the Blendtec and Vitamix have a 2+ peak horsepower motor. Any other blender will blend the tough

water. I was thinking, "I will just close my eyes and nose and drink it." But as soon as I opened the lid, I closed it again quickly because I felt queasy from the strong, wheatgrass smell. That dark green, almost black mixture was totally unconsumable. After some brainstorming, I added several bananas and blended it again. And that was when the magic began! I slowly, and with some trepidation, removed the lid and sniffed the air, and to my greatest surprise this bright green concoction smelled very pleasant. I cautiously tasted a sip and was exhilarated! It was better than tasty! Not too sweet, not too bitter, it was the most unusual taste I had ever tried, and I could describe it in one word: freshness.

In four hours I had consumed all I blended, which was one bunch of kale, four bananas and a quart of water. I felt wonderful and made more. Triumphantly, I realized that this evening was the first time in my life that I consumed two good-sized bunches of greens in one day. Plus, I ate them without any oil or salt! And I enjoyed the whole experience. My stomach felt fine and I was happy to have achieved my goal.

That was in August, 2004. The solution to my greens dilemma was so unexpectedly simple. To consume greens in this way took so little time that I naturally continued experimenting with blended greens and fruits day after day.

I must admit here, that the idea of blended greens was not new to me. Eleven years ago when my family was studying

---

cellulose of greens only so long as its blades are sharp. Unfortunately, when the blades become dull, they just move around pieces of banana and the blender very quickly overheats. Eleven years ago, after burning several blenders, I finally bought myself a Vitamix at the country fair. It still works like new.

at the Creative Health Institute (CHI) in Michigan, we were taught about the extraordinary healing properties of energy soup: blended sprouts, avocado, and apple. This soup was invented by Dr. Ann Wigmore, the pioneer of the Living Foods lifestyle in the 20th century. Although we were told countless times how exceptionally beneficial energy soup was, most of the guests at the institute were not able to eat more than a couple of spoonfuls of energy soup because it was not palatable.

I was very impressed with the testimonials that I heard from people about the benefits of energy soup. When I returned home I desperately experimented with energy soup, trying to improve the taste because I wanted my family to benefit from eating it. My final attempt to perfect energy soup was ended one day when I heard Valya yelling to Sergei in the back yard, "Run! Mom is making that green mush again!"

Despite all the evidence of the healing powers of energy soup, I found that unfortunately, even people who desperately needed and wanted it, could not make themselves consume it regularly.

I am amazed that eleven years after being introduced to energy soup, when I had completely forgotten all about it, I came back to the very same idea of blended greens from an entirely new direction. When I first started drinking green smoothies, I didn't mention it to anybody and did not expect anything significant to happen. Since I did not have any big health problems, I was not pursuing any dramatic changes. I just didn't want to age so noticeably. However, after about a month of erratic green smoothie drinking, two moles and a wart I had since early childhood peeled off my body. I felt more energized than ever before, and started sharing my experience with my family and friends. The next thing I noticed was that those cravings I had occasionally for heavy foods like nuts or crackers, especially in the evenings, had totally disappeared. I noticed that many of the wrinkles on my face went away and I began to hear compliments from other people about my fresh look. My nails became stronger, my vision sharpened and I had a wonderful taste in my mouth, even upon waking in the morning (pleasure I hadn't had since youth).

My dream had come true at last! I was consuming plenty of greens every day. I began to feel lighter and my energy increased. My tastes started to change. I discovered that my body was so starved for greens that for several weeks, I lived almost entirely on green smoothies. Plain fruits and vegetables became much more desirable for me and my cravings for fatty foods declined dramatically. I stopped consuming any kind of salt altogether, even seaweed.

Two weeks later, my husband and I were walking in California along a grassy trail when I suddenly began to salivate from looking at the dark green crispy branches of malva weeds growing in abundance along our path. I kept catching myself wanting to grab and eat them. I shared my observations with Igor and he listened attentively but didn't get excited. He had already noticed that I was eating differently lately. Instead of making myself a huge salad consisting of multiple chopped vegetables, a large avocado, sea salt, lots of onion and olive oil, I now chopped a bunch of lettuce with a tomato, sprinkled it with lemon juice and enjoyed it tremendously, rolling my eyes and humming with pleasure. I did not miss my former food, and felt completely satisfied eating so simply. Now I knew that the **human body can learn to crave greens!**

There was another change that astounded me. I used to have cravings for unhealthy foods when I got tired. For example, in the past, when we were traveling and we spent the night in an airplane, or after we were driving all night, I experienced severe cravings for some heavy raw foods or even some authentic Russian cooked foods from childhood that I hadn't eaten for more than a decade. These cravings were very strong and annoying. Driven by these urges, I would prepare myself some kind of dense raw food, like seed cheese with crackers, or stuff myself with nuts, sometimes late at night. I have heard from many other people that they experienced similar patterns. Also, during previous years, when I came home late from my office, often after ten p.m., I enjoyed changing my focus from work to other lighter topics, either by reading a chapter from a book or by watching a nice video. I noticed that if I allowed myself to grab an apple or a handful of nuts, I would tend to continue grazing and couldn't ever achieve a feeling of satisfaction. Even if I used my will power and didn't touch any food at home, I continued to feel discontent and food kept coming to my mind.

When I began to drink green smoothies, I noticed right away that those kinds of cravings disappeared. That was when my husband really noticed the difference in my behavior. In the evening after a hard work day, he would still crave something to eat while I was relaxed and content by just reading a book or talking. When Igor saw how happy I was in the evenings, along with the noticeable improvements in my health, he joined me in drinking green smoothies. He started to ask for a cup of "that green stuff" whenever I was making it.

Neither Igor nor I had any illnesses, so in the beginning it was hard to tell if we were just excited or if we really felt better. But soon both Igor and I were able to testify that we experienced rejuvenation and we began to look younger.

After only two months of drinking smoothies, Igor's mustache and beard started growing blacker, making him look like he did when we first met.

Igor became so enthusiastic about his youthful look that he became the green smoothie champion of my family. He would wake up early and make two or three gallons of smoothie every day: one for me, one for him, and one for Sergei and Valya to share. Both of our children enjoyed including this tasty green drink in their daily menu even though they were already experiencing great health. They noticed still more benefits, like the ability to sleep less, more complete eliminations, stronger nails, and most of all, improvement in their teeth, which became less sensitive.

One of my fears was that I would get tired of green smoothies one day, and I wouldn't want them any more. Yet, after six months of regular consumption I was enjoying them more than ever. Now I couldn't imagine my life without my green smoothies, as they had become 80% of my diet. In addition to smoothies, I ate flax crackers, salads, fruit and occasionally seeds or nuts. In order to always have the opportunity to make fresh green smoothie for myself, I purchased an additional Vitamix blender for my office. Whenever friends or customers came in, they saw a big green cup next to my computer and I treated them to a sample of my new discovery. To my great satisfaction, everybody loved it, despite their different dietary habits. Unexpectedly for me, some of my friends and coworkers started to comment on their health improvements just from the cup of green smoothie they were drinking in my office! No kidding! My web designer began to crave more raw foods as a result of rather irregular helpings of smoothies and lost 15 pounds in a couple of months. The woman from the office across the road got rid of her eczema by drinking a cup of green smoothie almost every day. Even the UPS guy liked it.

Inspired by the warm reception, I wrote an article "Ode to Green Smoothie" and emailed it to all those in my Internet address book. Almost instantly I began to receive strong, positive feedback and many detailed testimonials from my friends, students, and customers. While I felt compelled to do more research, it looked like the multiple benefits of green smoothie became obvious to everybody who tried them, and the number of people who were drinking green smoothie turned into a "green wave," growing rapidly every day.

CHAPTER FIVE

Why is it Hard to Love Greens?

*"Life expectancy would grow by leaps and bounds
if green vegetables smelled as good as bacon."*
DOUG LARSON

Green leaves were never included into our food pyramids as a separate group because humans never looked at them as real food. Carrot tops have several times more nutrition than the roots, but the opinion that greens are for rabbits, sheep, and cows, has been preventing us from eating carrot tops in our salads. We routinely throw away the most nutritious part of the carrot plant! The roots are much more palatable to human taste than the tops because the roots contain significantly more sugar and water. The tops are bitter from the abundant amount of nutrients in them.

The following charts (on pages 33–35) clearly show the nutritional supremacy of the leaves over the roots in three different plants: beets, parsley and turnips.[14] The only three categories in which roots are higher than leaves are calories, carbohydrates and sugar (except for turnips). These are the

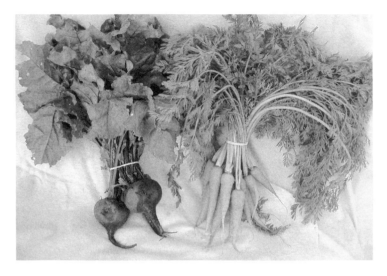

three components that make roots more palatable to us than the tops. I hope you will be impressed with some of these figures. For example, calcium in beet tops is 7 times higher than in its roots and vitamin A is 192 times higher in the tops than in the roots! In turnips vitamin K in the tops is 2,500 (!) times higher than in the roots. The compelling difference between nutrients in these two parts of the plants is obvious and indisputable. Think about thousands of tons of highly nutritious food, the green tops of the root vegetables, that are wasted year after year due to our ignorance, while the majority of people suffer from chronic deficiencies.

Naturally, one question comes to mind. **Why don't greens taste good to us?** Isn't our body wise enough to intuitively crave what it needs? Only few times in my life I have met people who have loved and craved greens. They told me that their parents didn't give them stimulating foods, such as candy or fried foods, when they were babies. I consider these friends of mine to be the luckiest people in the world. They are ecstatic

Nutritional Comparison of Roots and Greens

BEETS, 100 grams

Nutrients	Beets	Beet Greens
Calories	43.00	22.00
Protein (g)	1.61	2.20
Fat Total (g)	0.17	0.13
Carbohydrate (g)	9.56	4.33
Fiber – Total (g)	2.80	3.70
Sugar – Total (g)	6.76	0.50
Calcium (mg)	16.00	117.00
Iron (mg)	0.80	2.57
Magnesium (mg)	23.00	70.00
Phosphorus (mg)	40.00	41.00
Potassium (mg)	325.00	762.00
Sodium (mg)	78.00	226.00
Zinc (mg)	0.35	0.38
Copper (mg)	0.08	0.19
Manganese (mg)	0.33	0.39
Selenium (mg)	0.70	0.90
Vitamin C (mg)	4.90	30.00
Thiamin (mg)	0.03	0.10
Riboflavin (mg)	0.04	0.22
Niacin (mg)	0.33	0.40
Vitamin B6 (mg)	0.07	0.11
Folate – Total (mcg)	109.00	15.00
Food – Folate (mcg)	109.00	15.00
Folate – DFE (mcg_DEF)	109.00	15.00
Vitamin B12 (mcg)	0.00	0.00
Vitamin A (IU)	33.00	6326.00
Retinol (mcg)	0.00	0.00
Vitamin E (mg)	0.04	1.50
Vitamin K (mcg)	0.20	400.00
Fat – Saturated (g)	0.03	0.02
Fat – Monosaturated (g)	0.03	0.03
Fat – Polysaturated (g)	0.06	0.05
Cholesterol (mg)	0.0	0.00

Nutritional Comparison of Roots and Greens

PARSLEY, 100 grams

Nutrients	Parsnips (root)	Parsley
Calories	75.00	36.00
Protein (g)	1.20	2.97
Fat Total (g)	0.30	0.79
Carbohydrate (g)	17.99	6.33
Fiber – Total (g)	4.90	3.30
Sugar – Total (g)	4.80	0.85
Calcium (mg)	36.00	138.00
Iron (mg)	0.59	6.20
Magnesium (mg)	29.00	50.00
Phosphorus (mg)	71.00	58.00
Potassium (mg)	375.00	554.00
Sodium (mg)	10.00	56.00
Zinc (mg)	0.59	1.07
Copper (mg)	0.12	0.15
Manganese (mg)	0.56	0.16
Selenium (mg)	1.80	0.10
Vitamin C (mg)	17.00	133.00
Thiamin (mg)	0.09	0.09
Riboflavin (mg)	0.05	0.10
Niacin (mg)	0.70	1.31
Vitamin B6 (mg)	0.09	0.09
Folate – Total (mcg)	67.00	152.00
Food – Folate (mcg)	67.00	152.00
Folate – DFE (mcg_DEF)	67.00	152.00
Vitamin B12 (mcg)	0.00	0.00
Vitamin A (IU)	0.00	8424.00
Retinol (mcg)	0.00	0.00
Vitamin E (mg)	1.49	0.75
Vitamin K (mcg)	22.50	1640.00
Fat – Saturated (g)	0.05	0.13
Fat – Monosaturated (g)	0.11	0.29
Fat – Polysaturated (g)	0.05	0.12
Cholesterol (mg)	0.00	0.00

Nutritional Comparison of Roots and Greens

TURNIPS, 100 grams

Nutrients	Turnips	Turnip Greens
Calories	28.00	32.00
Protein (g)	0.90	1.50
Fat Total (g)	0.10	0.30
Carbohydrate (g)	6.43	7.13
Fiber – Total (g)	1.80	3.20
Sugar – Total (g)	3.80	0.81
Calcium (mg)	30.00	190.00
Iron (mg)	0.30	1.10
Magnesium (mg)	11.00	31.00
Phosphorus (mg)	27.00	42.00
Potassium (mg)	191.00	296.00
Sodium (mg)	67.00	40.00
Zinc (mg)	0.27	0.19
Copper (mg)	0.09	0.35
Manganese (mg)	0.13	0.47
Selenium (mg)	0.70	1.20
Vitamin C (mg)	21.00	60.00
Thiamin (mg)	0.04	0.07
Riboflavin (mg)	0.03	0.10
Niacin (mg)	0.40	0.60
Vitamin B6 (mg)	0.09	0.26
Folate – Total (mcg)	15.00	194.00
Food – Folate (mcg)	15.00	194.00
Folate – DFE (mcg_DEF)	15.00	194.00
Vitamin B12 (mcg)	0.00	0.00
Vitamin A (IU)	0.00	0.00
Retinol (mcg)	0.00	0.00
Vitamin E (mg)	0.03	2.86
Vitamin K (mcg)	0.10	251.00
Fat – Saturated (g)	0.01	0.07
Fat – Monosaturated (g)	0.01	0.02
Fat – Polysaturated (g)	0.05	0.12
Cholesterol (mg)	0.00	0.00

about a piece of cucumber or a fresh tomato. Looking at snow peas makes them salivate. My friend Vanessa says,

"Simple food has always tasted best to me. You really cannot appreciate the essence of a food unless you eat it all by itself. Then you can really enjoy its true taste. When my mom and I go to parties, we usually just eat the green leafy garnish from underneath the cuts of cheese. I would prefer it if the kale was on top of the cheese, but at least it's there."

However, most people would be distraught if they came to a party to find only cucumbers, tomatoes, and peas, or even worse, just that bed of greens. It seems clear to me that if we do crave the foods with stimulants, like sugar, caffeine, white flour, it means that our intricate bodily homeostasis has become distorted.

In the last few centuries, the human body has changed. The foods that have more stimulating tastes have become more appetizing to us than natural, unprocessed foods. However, everyone recognizes the reality that we cannot thrive on chocolate and pasta alone no matter how tasty they seem to be. From my research, I have learned that many people would not agree to a bland or bitter diet for the sake of feeling better even if they have a life threatening illness. Yet, many are continuing to inquire, "What are we supposed to eat? How are we supposed to feed our children in order to achieve better health?" Remarkably, green smoothies are not only nutritious, but also delightfully palatable even to children.

I strongly believe that it is possible to restore our ability to like and crave healthy foods. We could learn to live on a natural, healthy diet, even though we have developed some powerful, unnatural cravings.

CHAPTER SIX

Greens:
A New Food Group

I wonder how greens, such as kale, romaine lettuce, spinach, carrot tops, and others got classified as vegetables? Why do we call many completely different food groups *vegetables*, when they look different and contain different sets of nutrients? A produce manager from a local health food store complained to me that his customers often got confused when looking for a particular ingredient among 150+ pieces of produce all gathered under the single name: vegetables. This man had worked in the produce section for more than ten years. He suggested that the produce section be divided into several different smaller groups of plant foods with specific similarities, like roots (carrots, beets, daikon, etc.) flowers (broccoli, cauliflower, artichoke, etc.) and non-sweet fruit (cucumber, zucchini, squash, tomato, etc.). Combining foods with similar nutritional values would not only help shoppers to find necessary ingredients faster, but also would help them to become familiar with more plant foods and increase their variety of vegetarian food consumption.

Obviously, people have never considered plants to be important enough to be classified properly. Even at the regular supermarket one can see that other food departments have more detailed classifications. For example, the meat department is divided into poultry, fish, and meat, which in turn is subdivided into smaller sections, like veal, ground meats, bones, sub-products. Every item is carefully categorized, specifying which part of the carcass it is from. Cheeses have their own specification. Nobody would ever classify cheese and meat together in one group like "sandwich food," because it would be inconvenient and unclear. Yet this kind of confusion and error continually occurs in the produce section. Some errors are quite serious, to such a degree that they could cause health problems. As an example of this, placing starchy roots in the same category with tomatoes and rhubarb could prompt customers to make improper food combining choices. Many nutritionists believe in the benefits of proper food combining.[15] For example, starchy tubers combined in one meal with sour fruits or vegetables can create fermentation and gas in our intestines.

Placing greens in the same category as vegetables has caused people to mistakenly apply the combining rules of starchy vegetables to greens. Driven by this confusion, many concerned people wrote to me inquiring if blending fruits with greens was proper food combining. They had heard that "fruits and vegetables did not mix well." Yes, to combine starchy vegetables with fruits would not be a good idea. Such a combination can cause gas in the intestines. However, **greens are not vegetables** and greens are not starchy. In fact, greens are the only food group that helps digest other foods through stimulating the secretion of digestive enzymes. Thus, greens can be combined with any other foods. In addition, it has been recorded that chimpanzees often consume fruits and leaves off of the same tree at the same feeding time. In fact, Jane Goodall and other researchers have observed them rolling fruits inside of leaves and eating them as "sandwiches."

Yet, there is another great misconception which results from placing greens and vegetables into the same category. Such inappropriate generalizations have lead researchers to the erroneous conclusion that greens are a poor source of protein. Contrary to this popular belief, greens are an excellent source of protein, as you will see in the following chapter.

I propose that we separate greens from vegetables, now and forevermore. Greens have never received proper attention and have never been researched adequately because they have been incorrectly identified as vegetables. We don't even have a proper name for greens in most languages. The name "dark green leafy vegetables" is long and inconvenient to use, similar to "the animal with horns that gives milk."

We don't have complete nutritional data about greens. For this book I had to collect bits and pieces of information out of books and magazines from different countries and I still don't have all the parts. I have not, for example, been able to find the complete nutritional content of carrot tops anywhere. Nevertheless, I have enough to draw some essential conclusions: **greens are the primary food group that match human nutritional needs most completely.**

In the following chart please see a list of all essential minerals and vitamins that are recommended by USDA and a list of these nutrients available in Kale and Lambsquarters (an edible weed). Based on this data, we can conclude that greens are the most essential food for humans.

Essential Mineral and Vitamin Content

LAMBSQUARTERS (a weed) and KALE

Nutrients Adequate Intake or RDA[16]	Kale One pound raw	Lambsquarters (weed) One pound raw
Folic Acid – 400 mcg/day	132 mcg	136.0 mcg
Niacin – 16 mg/day	4.8 mg	5.4 mg
Pantothenic Acid – 5 mg/day	0.68 mg	0.45 mg
Riboflavin (B2) – 1.3 mg/day	0.68 mg	0.9 mg
Thiamin (B1) – 1.2 mg/day	0.68 mg	1.8 mg
Vitamin A – 900 mcg/day	21,012.0 mcg	15,800.0 mcg
Vitamin B6 – 1.3 mg/day	68.0 mg	8.0 mg
Vitamin B12 – 2.4 mcg/day	data unavailable	data unavailable
Vitamin C – 90 mg/day	547.0 mg	363.0 mg
Vitamin D – 5 mcg/day (based on absence of adequate exposure to sunlight)*	data unavailable See note	data unavailable See note
Vitamin E – 15 mg/day	data unavailable	data unavailable
Vitamin K – 120 mcg/day	3,720.0 mcg	data unavailable

Minerals

Calcium – 1,000 mg/day	615.0 mg	1403.0 mg
Iron – 10 mg/day	7.5 mg	5.4 mg
Magnesium – 400 mg/day	155.0 mg	154.0 mg
Phosphorus – 700 mg/day	255.0 mg	327.0 mg
Potassium – 4.7 g/day	2.1 g	2.1 g
Sodium – 1.5 g/day	0.2 g	0.2 g
Zinc – 15 mg/day	2.0 mg	1.8 mg
Copper 1.5 mg/day	1.4 mg	1.4 mg
Manganese 10 mg/day	3.4 mg	3.6 mg
Selenium – 70 mcg/day	4.0 mcg	4.1 mcg

*For a caucasian with medium skin pigmentation, exposure of the face, hands, and arms for five minutes two or three times a week for three-fourths of the year actually eliminates the need for dietary intake of vitamin D.

CHAPTER SEVEN

Abundance of Proteins in Greens

"I submit that scientists have not yet explored the hidden possibilities of the innumerable seeds, leaves and fruits for giving the fullest possible nutrition to mankind."
MAHATMA GANDHI

*E*very protein molecule consists of a chain of amino acids. An **essential amino acid** is one that cannot be synthesized by the body, and therefore must be supplied as part of the diet. Humans must include adequate amounts of 9 amino acids in their diet.

Professor T. Colin Campbell shows in his book, *The China Study*, that the U.S. RDA for protein is greatly overestimated. Studies of the diets of chimpanzees compared to that of humans confirm the same truth. "Chimpanzees maintain a fairly low and constant protein intake, due to their focus on fruit . . ."[17]

I have looked at the nutritional content of dozens of various green vegetables and I was pleased to see that the aminos that were low in one plant were high in another. In other words, if we maintain a variety of greens in our diet, we will cover all essential aminos in abundance.

Please look at the chart of the essential amino acid content in kale and lambsquarters. I have chosen kale because it is available in most produce markets. Lambsquarters is one of the most common edible weeds that grows in different climates. Most farmers should be able to identify lambsquarters for you.

In the left hand column you see the recommended amounts of essential amino acids for an average adult.[18] In the right column you can see the amounts of those amino acids contained in lambsquarters and kale. Please notice that dark green leafy vegetables contain similar or larger amounts of amino acids than the Recommended Daily Allowance (RDA).

As you can see from this chart, one pound of kale has even more protein than is recommended by the USDA per day. Yet, by erroneously placing all parts of plants (roots, stalks, blossoms, spears, greens, etc.) into the category of vegetables, and assuming they have the same properties, we have mistakenly concluded that greens are a poor source of protein. This inaccurate conclusion has led to the malnourishment and suffering of people for decades. The lack of research on the nutritional content of greens has led to a great confusion among the majority of people, including many professionals. Dr. Joel Fuhrman wrote in his book *Eat to Live*: "Even physicians and dietitians ... are surprised to learn that ... when you eat large quantities of green vegetables, you receive a considerable amount of protein."

Where do I get my protein? Being aware of the confusion around vegetables, I understand why this became a popular

Essential Amino Acid Content

LAMBSQUARTERS (a weed) and KALE

AMINO ACIDS	RDA for average adult (mg/day)	Content (mg) in LAMBSQUARTERS One pound raw
Histidine	560	527
Isoleucine	700	1149
Leucine	980	1589
Lysine	840	1607
Methionine + cystine	910	222 + 404 = 626
Phenylalanine + tyrosine	980	754 + 795 = 1549
Threonine	490	740
Tryptophan	245	173
Valine	700	1026

AMINO ACIDS	RDA for average adult (mg/day)	Content (mg) in KALE One pound raw
Histidine	560	313
Isoleucine	700	895
Leucine	980	1051
Lysine	840	895
Methionine + cystine	910	145 + 200 = 345
Phenylalanine + tyrosine	980	766 + 532 = 1298
Threonine	490	668
Tryptophan	245	182
Valine	700	820

question. Since most people were not aware that greens have an abundance of readily available essential amino acids, they were trying to eat from the other food groups known for their rich protein content. However, let me explain the difference between complex proteins found in meat, dairy, fish, etc. and individual amino acids, found in fruits, vegetables, and especially in greens.

It is clear that the body has to work a lot less when creating protein from the assortment of individual amino acids from greens, rather than the already combined, long molecules of protein, assembled according to the foreign pattern of a totally different creature such as a cow or a chicken. I would like to explain the difference between complex proteins and individual amino acids with a simple anecdote.

Imagine that you have to make a wedding dress for your daughter. Consuming the complex proteins that we get from cows or other creatures is like going to the second hand store, and buying many other people's used dresses, coming home and spending several hours ripping apart pieces of the dresses that you like and combining them into a new dress for your daughter. This alternative will take a lot of time and energy and will leave a great deal of garbage. You could never make a perfect dress this way.

Consuming individual amino acids is like taking your daughter to a fabric store to buy beautiful new fabric, lace, buttons, ribbons, threads, and pearls. With these essential elements you can make a beautiful dress that fits her unique body perfectly. Similarly, when you eat greens, you "purchase" new amino acids, freshly made by sunshine and chlorophyll, which the body will use to rebuild its parts according to your own unique DNA.

Contrary to this, your body would have a hard time trying to make a perfect molecule of protein out of someone else's molecules, which consist of totally different combinations of amino acids. Plus, your body would most likely receive a lot of unnecessary pieces that are hard to digest. These pieces would be floating around in your blood like garbage for a long time, causing allergies and other health problems. Professor W. A. Walker from the Department of Nutrition at the Harvard School of Public Health, states that, "Incompletely digested protein fragments may be absorbed into the bloodstream. The absorption of these large molecules contributes to the development of food allergies and immunological disorders."[19]

The ironic result of consuming this imperfect source of protein, (animal protein), is that many people develop deficiencies in essential amino acids. Such deficiencies are not only dangerous to health, but they dramatically change people's perceptions of life and the way people feel and behave. The body in producing neurotransmitters uses some essential amino acids, like tyrosine, tryptophan, glutamine, histamine, and others. Neurotransmitters are the natural chemicals that facilitate communication between brain cells. These substances govern our emotions, memory, moods, behavior, learning abilities and sleep patterns. For the last three decades, neurotransmitters have been the focus of mental health research.

According to the research of Julia Ross, a specialist in nutritional psychology,[20] if your body lacks certain amino acids, you may develop strong symptoms of mental and physiological imbalance and severe cravings for unwanted substances.

For example, let us consider tyrosine and phenylalanine. The symptoms of a deficiency in these amino acids can cause:

- Depression
- Lack of energy
- Lack of focus and concentration
- Attention deficit disorder

In addition, the symptoms of a deficiency in these amino acids may lead to cravings for:

- ❀ Sweets   ❀ Aspartame   ❀ Caffeine
- ❀ Starch   ❀ Alcohol   ❀ Cocaine
- ❀ Chocolate   ❀ Marijuana   ❀ Tobacco

Using available data from official sources [21] I have calculated the amounts of these two essential amino acids that we can receive from either chicken or dark green endive:

CHICKEN One serving:	ENDIVE One head:
222 mg tyrosine	205 mg tyrosine
261 mg phenylalanine	272 mg phenylalanine

As you can see, contrary to the popular opinion, there are plenty of high quality proteins in greens. According to the explanation of Professor T. Colin Campbell, "There is a mountain of compelling evidence showing that so called "low-quality" plant protein, which allows for slow but steady synthesis of new proteins, is the healthiest type of protein." [22] For example, the protein from greens doesn't have cancer as a side effect. Yet, in many books, greens are not even listed as a protein source because greens have not been researched enough.

Greens have sufficient protein to build muscle in grazing animals. I received this testimony from my very first American friend, a farmer with a BA in psychology from Harvard University, Peter Hagerty of Maine: "When our sheep are in the barn eating *concentrated feed* such as ground corn and oats, they gain weight much more *quickly*, but young lambs, once they reach 120 lbs or 90 % of slaughter weight, begin putting this concentrated food into *fat* rather than muscle which is not advantageous for the consumer who has to trim this fat off and throw it away. If the lambs are *grass fed*, they grow more *slowly* but they can reach full slaughter weight with *very little fat*. So my observations are: concentrates seem to put on easily burnable fats and grasses put on quality muscle."

In summary, greens provide protein in the form of individual amino acids. These amino acids are easier for the body to utilize than complex proteins. A variety of greens can supply all the protein we need to sustain each of our unique bodies.

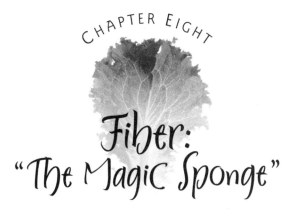

CHAPTER EIGHT

Fiber: "The Magic Sponge"

*D*r. Bernard Jensen, D.C., Ph.D., one of the most renowned nutrition experts in the world and author of many popular health books, stated that:

> "Any cleansing program should begin in the colon ... In the 50 years I've spent helping people to overcome illness, disability and disease, it has become crystal clear that poor bowel management lies at the root of most people's health problems. In treating over 300,000 patients, it is the bowel that invariably has to be cared for first before any effective healing can take place."[23]

The main purpose of consuming fiber is elimination. **Without fiber, complete elimination is nearly impossible, if possible at all.** The human body is built miraculously in such a way that almost all the toxins from every part of the body, including millions of dead cells, end up in the human sewage system daily — the colon. The colon fills up with waste matter so full of poison that we look at it with disgust, not daring to touch it. In order to eliminate this matter, the body needs fiber.

There are two main kinds of fiber: soluble and insoluble. Soluble fiber is found in fruit, beans, peas, oat bran and especially in chia seeds. It has a gel-like consistency that improves bowel movements by increasing the volume of bulk in the colon. Soluble fiber binds together cholesterol in the small intestines and takes it out of the body. Certain soluble fibers such as pectin (found in apples) and guar gums (found in chia seed, oatmeal, legumes and mangos) slow down the release of the sugars contained in the foods we eat, thus reducing the risk of diabetes.

Insoluble fiber is found primarily in greens, peels, nuts, seeds, beans and skins of grains. The elimination system is very complex. It has been perfected by nature to every minute action. I'll try to explain this complicated process with a very simple example. Insoluble fiber under a microscope looks like a sponge, and indeed it serves us as a miraculous sponge, because every piece of it can absorb many times more toxins than its own volume. Have you ever wondered why we always like to have a sponge in our kitchen? We never use something smooth, like paper or plastic to wipe dirty counters clean. Sponges are fibrous. They make the job of cleaning easier by absorbing dirt. So does insoluble fiber. It grabs the toxins and takes them out of the body and into the toilet. Insoluble fiber is much better than any sponge because it can hold several times more toxins than its own size. I call it a magic sponge.

If we do not consume fiber, most of the toxic waste accumulates in our body. Our body is constructed in such a marvelous way that all the toxins are directed to the bowels. This is the human body's sewage system. We need to understand that we have to eliminate many pounds of toxins regularly.

Where do toxins come from? They come not only from inhaling dust and asbestos, undigested food, ingested heavy metals and pesticides. A large amount of toxins come from the dead cells of our own bodies. We know that cells are tiny and sometimes conclude that the cell could not add much to the amount of waste in our body. However, let's keep in mind that every year as much as 98% of the total number of atoms in our body are replaced.[24] That means anywhere from 70–100 pounds of dead cells per year, or more, should be passing out of our system. If they don't, the dead cells of our own body can be one of the most toxic kinds of waste because they begin to rot right away. It is important to understand that when we do not consume enough fiber, we accumulate a lot more waste than our bodies can handle.

Just as one cannot clean a kitchen without a sponge, the human body cannot eliminate without fiber. Picture yourself being challenged to clean some large, dirty space like a garage, with nothing but plastic wrap. I would give up. The human body won't give up, but if there is no fiber, the first thing that happens is our skin tries to take on the elimination "job" and as a result the skin becomes rough and bumpy. When our bowels are clogged, our body attempts to excrete more mucus, through our eyes, nose, and throat, we sweat a lot more — the body uses every possible channel to eliminate, but it's like pushing the garbage out through the window screen instead of the door. By consuming enough insoluble fiber we unlock the door to eliminate toxins from the body the easy and normal way.

Now you are probably wondering how much fiber we need to consume for optimal health benefits. According to research, the average wild chimpanzee consumes 300 grams of fiber per day![25] When I read that, I calculated how much fiber I consumed each day. I came up with only 3 grams, because I used to love juicing. Very often I would juice my fruits and vegetables rather than "waste" my time and effort on chewing them. About thirty years ago, in the first books about juicing I read, I learned that fiber was not digestible, contained no nutrients, and served merely as a strain on the human intestinal tract. Since then juicing became one of my regular habits. I was proudly juicing for days, even weeks, trying to "cleanse" myself of toxins, and I considered myself to be maintaining a very healthy diet! I became astounded by the comparison of 300 grams with three. Moreover, I realized how harmful it was for my health when I consumed zero fiber by juicing all the time. I decided that I couldn't afford to throw my fiber in the compost any more. Green smoothies are definitely superior to juices. Yet I still consider that juicing could contribute to health in specific situations.

Albert Mosseri, famous French doctor of Natural Hygiene, has radically changed the classical "Sheltonian" method of fasting on water. After supervising 4,000 long-term water fasts conducted at his clinic, he came to the extraordinary conclusion that long-term fasts were a "risky waste of time." He now oversees much shorter water fasts followed by what he calls "half-fasts," in which he introduces a limited amount of food rich in fiber in addition to water. During this important stage of healing, his patients receive only one pound of fruits and one pound of vegetables daily until their elimination is complete.[26] Dr. Mosseri states that switching to this "half-fast" method has accelerated elimination to such a degree that 100% of his patients develop profound signs of a deep cleansing process in the form of a dark coating of their tongue, often charcoal black or dark brown.

Massive amounts of research on dietary fiber have been done all around the world since the beginning of the last century. We now have tons of undeniable evidence of fiber's many healing properties. Here are some of them:

- Fiber can strengthen a diseased heart.[27]
- Fiber reduces cholesterol which decreases the risk of heart disease.
- Fiber prevents many different kinds of cancer, reduces cancer risks and binds carcinogens.
- Fiber can lessen the risk of diabetes and improve already diagnosed diabetes.
- Fiber steadies blood-sugar levels by slowing down the absorption of sugar.[28]
- Fiber can strengthen the immune system.
- Fiber keeps our bowels healthy, relieves constipation, and promotes regularity.
- Fiber prevents gallstones.[29]
- Fiber promotes healthy intestinal bacteria.
- Fiber helps us lose weight and curbs overeating.
- Fiber binds up excess estrogen.
- Fiber prevents ulcers.

The U.S. recommended daily allowance for fiber is 30 grams per day. The average American consumes between 10 and 15 grams of fiber per day.[30] That is far from sufficient. Considering the fact that these 10 tiny grams of fiber would have to absorb and move out several huge pounds of waste matter, 10 grams is almost nothing. I think insufficient fiber intake is the main reason for aging in humans. Look at any animal that lives in the wild. One can hardly guess the age of a deer, zebra, eagle or giraffe. Whether they are at the age of two or fifteen years old, they look the same. Wild animals only begin to slow down during the last weeks before they die. On the other hand, it is often easy to guess the age of humans, down to five years. At the same time, I have seen many people who looked younger upon improving their elimination.

I believe we should consume 50 to 70 grams of fiber per day or more. However, **we have to increase the intake of fiber gradually. It can be dangerous to switch overnight from 10 grams to 70.**

Many of our bodies have degenerated over the decades due to the consumption of processed foods. In addition, we have adopted many unnatural practices like lack of exercise and spending most of the time indoors. Therefore, we need to reintroduce healthy habits into our life slowly to give our body time to readjust. Green smoothies are perfect for this gradual shift. Other sources of fiber and especially fiber in the pill form can often create too drastic of an increase of fiber in one's diet too fast and can result in a bloated feeling and increased gas. Such unpleasant side effects can cause people to give up before they even get a chance to experience the health benefits of fiber.

Fiber is an important component in the diets of chimpanzees. As I noted, they consume 300 grams of fiber per day. In addition to eating many fiber-rich fruits and leaves, they supplement their diet with pith and bark, both of which consist of approximately 44% fiber.

Flaxseed is a perfect addition to the human diet. Flaxseed is very high in both soluble fiber and insoluble fiber. It contains 26% fiber (14% soluble, 12% insoluble). Just ⅛ cup of flaxseed contains 6 grams of fiber.

I recommend adding flaxseed to your diet regularly. Flaxseeds have a tough outer coating and should be freshly ground in order to receive the most nutritional benefit. You can grind whole seeds with a coffee grinder or in a Vita Mix dry container. I recommend adding one or two tablespoons of ground flax meal to your salads, soups or smoothies. Flaxseed is also a good source of omega-3 fatty acids, and it is by far nature's richest source of plant lignin, an important anti-cancer phytonutrient.

My family has been intuitively adding flaxseed to our meals every day either in the form of crackers or as flax meal. Igor has perfected a method for dehydrating flax crackers to such a degree that he knows how to make his crackers taste like pumpernickel, or sourdough toast, or everyone's favorite Russian caraway bread. If you learn to make crackers like Igor, you will never be lonely and you will have plenty of fiber, nature's sponge, in your diet.

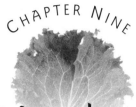

CHAPTER NINE

Greens for Homeostasis

"Look at this body! It's a work of art. No improvements can be made... divinely put together."
DR. BERNARD JENSEN[31]

The main difference between living things and non-living things is that living entities can repair themselves and thus adapt to the changes of the environment to a great extent, while the things that are not alive can get broken and destroyed. For example, if you tear a leaf off of a plant, it can grow a new leaf. If you cut the skin on your finger, your skin will heal itself. Alternatively, non-living things like rocks or man-made constructions, no matter how big and strong, if damaged can not repair themselves. For instance, after catastrophes like earthquakes, avalanches, and tornados people have to rebuild their homes, roads, power plants, etc.

This extraordinary ability of all living organisms to repair themselves is the only power that can heal any illness. All other healing techniques invented by people can be successful only if they are directed towards helping the body's own natural ability to regulate itself. A human body can heal a disease only when all bodily substances such as

57

lymph, blood, hormones, and countless others are maintained within particular optimal parameters.

A physiological process that keeps all substances in the body at the levels necessary for optimal body health is called homeostasis.[32] This process is extremely complex and the complete understanding of its mechanism goes far beyond our three-dimensional imagination. We are grateful to recognize that homeostasis is the most important process in the body. The simple truth is: **if we are helping our homeostasis — we are taking the best possible care of our health.**

How can we take care of our homeostasis when it is out of our reach? The process of homeostasis in the human body is tightly connected to the endocrine system. Homeostatic balance depends on the performance of the endocrine glands. If the glands do not secrete the proper amount of hormones, the homeostatic balance in the body will shift and disease could start.

The glands of the endocrine system and the hormones they release influence almost every cell, organ, and function of our body. The endocrine system is instrumental in regulating mood, growth and development, tissue function, and metabolism, as well as sexual function, and reproductive processes.

To make it really simple, the endocrine system in a human body acts like a factory combined with a supermarket that manufactures and supplies every substance requested by any gland or organ at any time, in any needed quantity. What would such factory need? An abundance of high quality supplies! Similarly, the endocrine system in our body absolutely needs all nutrients, including vitamins, amino acids, carbohydrates, essential fatty acids, minerals and all trace elements. Supplying all of these nutrients to our body is critical for good health.

Greens match all of these purposes better than any other food! Once again, when blended, the nutrients from greens are absorbed more efficiently and provide many times more nutrients than other foods and even traditionally made salads. In other words, **by drinking green smoothies we support our homeostatic balance in the most optimal way.**

I wish I knew this information ten years ago when my mother was still alive. She was only 66, a beautiful, adventurous woman, when she was diagnosed with cancer one year after she swam in the river near Chernobyl. I could have explained to her now very clearly how the body can heal. I am sure that Mom would have refused chemotherapy because those poisonous chemicals ruined her already weakened homeostasis. I would have nourished her to health instead. I understand now that only supporting (not destroying) the homeostasis gives a body the greatest chance to heal. She might still be with us. I have met many people who have survived cancers much more severe than what my mother had by incorporating more greens into their diet. I miss her. She knew how to share joy like no one else.

When older people come to my classes, I feel grateful that I have an opportunity to share my information with someone else's parents. I feel so happy for their children. What a blessing to have open-minded parents! I am trying hard to be one myself.

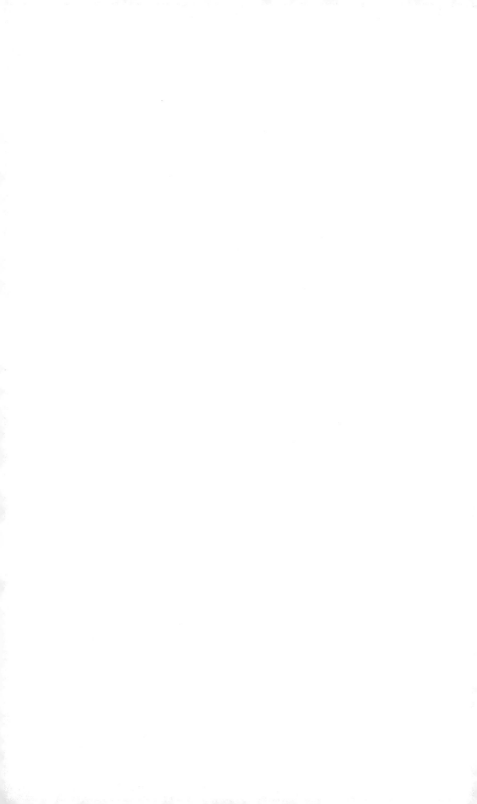

CHAPTER TEN

The Significance of Stomach Acid

How many people know what their measurement of stomach acid is? How many of us appreciate its importance for our overall health? Almost nobody recognizes how crucial it is to have normal hydrochloric acid in the stomach. I don't know why none of the many doctors I have ever visited have asked me about my hydrochloric acid, or tested it for me. I've never heard my friends talk about their stomach acid. I was grateful to learn about its importance from a veterinarian, who was helping me create a healthy diet for my dog.

To my surprise, I found scores of books and scientific articles about the connection between the level of hydrochloric acid and human health. This topic has been studied for decades. Professor W. A. Walker from the Department of Nutrition at the Harvard School of Public Health, states that, "Medical researchers since the 1930s have been concerned about the consequences of hypochlorhydria. While all the health consequences are still not entirely clear, some have been well documented."[33]

Low stomach acidity (hypochlorhydria) is a condition that occurs when the human body is unable to produce adequate quantities of stomach acid. Low stomach acidity inevitably and dramatically impacts digestion and absorption of most nutrients necessary for health. Most minerals, including such important ones as iron, zinc, calcium, and the B-complex vitamins (folic acid and others) need certain amounts of stomach acids *in order to be absorbed at all.* **Without stomach acid, nutritional deficiencies inevitably develop leading to disease.**

Besides absorption, stomach acid has many other important functions. For instance, stomach acid is supposed to destroy all harmful microorganisms, pathogenic bacteria, parasites and their eggs, and fungi that enter the body through the mouth. Therefore, **if stomach acid is insufficient, there is no barrier against parasites**. I have spoken with a gastroenterologist who takes test samples of stomach acid from his patients and often finds several kinds of parasites flourishing in the very place where they are supposed to be killed. I would want my stomach acid to be strong for this reason alone.

Stomach acid helps to digest large protein molecules.[34] If stomach acid is low, then incompletely digested protein fragments get absorbed into the bloodstream and cause allergies and immunological disorders.

The natural level of hydrochloric acid (HCl) decreases as we age, especially after the age of forty. That is when most people begin to develop gray hair as a result of nutritional deficiencies caused by lowered stomach acid. Hydrochloric acid could also start decreasing early in life if we abuse our gastrointestinal tract, or entire body, through food excesses, chemical use, and stress. Overeating, especially overconsumption of fats and proteins, wears out the parietal cells of the stomach that secret HCl.[35]

Indigenous people have had many different diets throughout history, depending on their environment. What they had in common was that they ate large amounts of fiber. Researchers have estimated that Australopithecus and some other indigenous people consumed roughly 150 grams of fiber daily.[36] By looking at this number, it's easy to suggest that the acidity of their stomachs was quite strong, a lot stronger than ours. They also had much stronger teeth, jaws, and jaw muscles. They were able to chew this rough, stringy food to a creamy consistency in their mouths, and then their stomachs continued digesting this well chewed matter by applying hydrochloric acid. Our bodies have dramatically changed since then. Make an experiment: take a piece of any vegetable or green leaf, sit down and chew it as long as you can. Just before you are ready to swallow it, spit it out onto your palm and take a look at it. You will see that it will still be far from a creamy consistency. Keep in mind that your body would only be able to assimilate nutrients from the tiniest particles. Large particles won't get digested and will turn into acidic waste. A friend of mine who is a doctor, and frequently takes blood tests, has shown me on a screen connected to a microscope such an undigested piece in the blood of a vegan patient. I was shocked to see that whenever this tiny undigested piece touched red blood cells, those cells instantly died. Eventually this piece of undigested food ended up being encircled in several layers of about a hundred dead cells. My friend explained to me that such toxic pieces accumulate in our small intestines causing people to have enlarged, protruding bellies.

If, in addition to improper chewing, some of us do not have the necessary concentration of hydrochloric acid, then it is very likely that a few of us have multiple nutritional deficiencies. In order to produce hydrochloric acid, the human body has to work very hard. As we grow older, our body becomes weaker and cannot produce adequate amounts of hydrochloric acid. That is why most people have less stomach acid as they age.

As we grow older, we develop gray hair. I have observed that most people diagnosed with very low stomach acid had noticeably more gray hair, which is an indirect sign of nutrient deficiencies. On the other hand, there are numerous well-documented accounts of people's natural hair color returning as a result of consuming blended greens on a regular basis, Ann Wigmore being one of them.

Blending is similar to chewing, therefore, eating blended food can make a dramatic improvement to our health. After being broken down in a high-speed blender, pieces of food become the perfect size for assimilation. As a result, the body doesn't keep the food in the stomach as long but sends it right into the small intestines, allowing the body to produce less hydrochloric acid. Consequently, **consuming blended foods saves us energy and keeps us youthful despite of aging.**

For many years I couldn't understand why some people quickly loose too much weight on a raw food diet. These people simply cannot stay on a raw food diet because they feel uncomfortable living their lives with constant remarks from their friends and relatives about being too thin. I agree that humans shouldn't be too skinny. After doing a lot of research about the impact of hypochlorhydria on assimilation of food, I asked some of my friends with this weight problem if they had ever checked their stomach acid level. Several of them got back to me and reported that they were diagnosed with very low or no stomach acid at all. Their doctor prescribed HCL pills to take with their meals. A close friend has been trying to eat raw for several years and became so thin that her husband became concerned for her health. She went to a doctor and was diagnosed with achlorhydria (no stomach acid). Her doctor put her on HCL pills and she continued her raw food diet. My friend gained *all* her weight back.

In order for nutrients to be absorbed, the food has to be broken in the stomach, both mechanically and with acids, into very small pieces of 1–2 mm. Raw fruits and vegetables have the most valuable nutrients in them, but they are especially hard to digest because their tough cellulose structure has to be ruptured in order to get all the nutrients out. If there is not enough stomach acid, the body is unable to receive all needed nutrients, especially proteins, and deficiencies start to develop. I have encountered several people with such a problem who felt as if they were trapped. While eating only raw food they were able to eliminate symptoms of certain illnesses that they had, but they became very skinny. Then they would add cooked food to their diet to gain their desired weight, but their unwanted symptoms would return. Puzzled, they kept going back and forth not knowing what to do.

That is why I felt great joy when, after teaching a couple of classes about green smoothies, I began receiving letters like this one:

> "Though the raw food took care of my arthritis I was never able to stick to it longer than two months because on raw foods alone, I dropped weight so quickly, down to 135 lbs, that my wife panicked thinking that I was dying, so I had to go back to cooked foods which made my arthritis return. When I started drinking green smoothies, my weight stabilized! I have been raw now for six months and keep my normal weight of 155 lbs. Thank you!" (N. H., Canada)

I have already witnessed many cases in which people with digestive problems were able to greatly improve their assimilation by adding blended greens to their diets. While cooking makes the food softer and easier to digest, in the process of heating, most essential vitamins and enzymes in the food get destroyed. Blending is a lot less harmful than cooking because it saves all the vital nutrients in the food.

There are numerous conditions that are associated with low stomach acidity.[37] These are just some of them: bacterial overgrowth, chronic candidacies, parasites, Addison's disease, multiple sclerosis, arthritis, asthma, auto immune disorders, celiac disease, stomach carcinoma, depression, dermatitis, diabetes, eczema, flatulence, gall bladder disease, gastric polyps, gastritis, hepatitis, hyperthyroidism, myasthenia gravis, osteoporosis, psoriasis, rosacea, ulcerative colitis, urticaria, and vitiligo. This is why the famous researcher, Dr. Theodore A. Baroody, stated in his wonderful book *Alkalize or Die,* "Hydrochloric acid is absolutely essential for life."[38] In other words, **no one can be completely healthy without normal hydrochloric acid.**

Please do not confuse acidity in the stomach with alkalinity of the blood. Our blood must be slightly alkaline and we will discuss it in up-coming chapters. "Hydrochloric acid is the *only* acid that our body produces. All other acids are by-products of metabolism and are eliminated as soon as possible."[39]

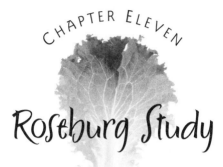

CHAPTER ELEVEN

Roseburg Study

When I became aware of the important functions of hydrochloric acid, I decided to perform a study. Based on the symptoms of low stomach acid that I gathered from different medical articles, I created the following questionnaire. I then printed a thousand copies and distributed them among my students. The results were shocking! I have calculated that 98.5% of people who answered my questionnaire had some symptoms of low stomach acidity. I invite you to check if you might have any indications of hypochlorhydria yourself.

SIGNS AND SYMPTOMS OF LOW STOMACH ACIDITY
Please read the question and check the appropriate box on the right

	NEVER	SOMETIMES	FREQUENTLY
Do you have bloating, belching or flatulence immediately after meals?	☐	☐	☐
Do you have indigestion, diarrhea, or constipation?	☐	☐	☐
Do you feel soreness, burning, or dryness of the mouth?	☐	☐	☐

	NEVER	SOMETIMES	FREQUENTLY
Do you have heartburn?	☐	☐	☐
Do you have multiple food allergies?	☐	☐	☐
Do you feel nauseous after taking supplements?	☐	☐	☐
Do you experience rectal itching?	☐	☐	☐
Do you have weak, peeling, and/or cracked fingernails?	☐	☐	☐
Do you have redness or dilated blood vessels in the cheeks and nose?	☐	☐	☐
Do you have adult acne?	☐	☐	☐
This question is only for women: do you experience hair loss?	☐	☐	☐
Do you have an iron deficiency?	☐	☐	☐
Do you have undigested food in the stools?	☐	☐	☐
Do you have chronic yeast infections?	☐	☐	☐
Do you have low tolerances for dentures?	☐	☐	☐

These symptoms can be indicators of hypochlorhydria. If you have marked several symptoms even in the "sometimes" column, you may want to check your stomach acidity at the doctor's office.

I spoke to a medical doctor from Russia and was intrigued to discover how they test hypochlorhydria there. They ask people to drink a quarter cup of beet juice and watch to see if the color of their stool or urine changes even slightly to the color of a beet. Now watch out! If it changes, then yes, your stomach acid is low. I was so amazed at this, because I believed that such a change of color is normal for everyone, as it always was for me. However, a few months after drinking green smoothies, my family ate a big delicious beet salad and none of us had a change in color anymore! Since I could only attribute such a dramatic change to drinking green smoothies, I assumed that our hydrochloric acid level had improved. In order to obtain more solid proof of this, I began planning a study that would show the effect of green smoothie on stomach acid. I wanted to find several people who were diagnosed with low hydrochloric acid and would volunteer to add green smoothies to their diets for a duration of time. After they completed drinking smoothies for a certain amount of time, they would be tested again.

By some magical coincidence, as I was praying to find a doctor who would be willing to help me with such a study, one sunny morning a physician named Dr. Paul Fieber called me from Roseburg, a nearby town in Oregon. He told me that he and his wife had recently adopted the raw food lifestyle and needed guidance. He also shared that recently he became disturbed by the fact that a great number of people had low stomach acid. We met the next morning to discuss our experiment in detail. Dr. Fieber seemed very interested in participating. The following week, Igor and I drove 120 miles to Roseburg to teach a nutrition class. After my lecture, 27 people stepped forward and offered to volunteer to drink one quart of freshly made green smoothies each day in addition to their regular mainstream American diet for one month.

This project started on April 29th 2005. My whole family took turns blending many gallons of the green drink. To increase variety, we used any fruits and greens we could get a hold of. Igor drove the valuable load 240 miles round trip, every other day. It was quite a commitment, not only for my family, but also for all the participating people and even their families. None of my dear participants ever missed a day to come to the pick up site. When I thanked this new family of mine (I call them "my in-raws") for being so dedicated and disciplined, they replied that they all felt the urgent importance of this experiment and were excited to help. Besides, many of them wanted to improve their stomach condition by natural means.

The following segment describes Dr. Fieber's side of the story.

DR. PAUL'S STORY

Meeting Victoria and her family was a wonderful experience. It was amazing how fate brought us together. My wife and I were looking for help on our path to improve our health through raw food and Victoria needed help with her study.

There are different methods of testing HCL, but we decided that the HCL challenge test would work out best for us, considering our time line. The HCL challenge test is designed to help determine the ability of the stomach to produce adequate stomach acid. The body has evolved to release stomach acid in response to appropriate stimuli. Thinking about food, chewing and the presence of certain foods (healthy or not) in the stomach e.g. proteins, milk, calcium salts, coffee . . . stimulate the release of Gastrin, a hormone secreted by Gastrin cells, or G cells, in the pyloric glands located in the antrum of the stomach. Gastrin strongly stimulates the parietal glands to produce and secrete acid into the stomach. Histamine is another hormone that stimulates acid production. Its effect is potentiated by the presence of Gastrin. Many people have a deficient acid-producing process and suffer from hypochlorhydria or in more serious cases achlorhydria.

Many of my patients complain of gastric reflux due to "excess" stomach acid secretion. In my experience, hypersecretion of stomach acid is not common. Inappropriate timing of stomach acid however is common, and can produce symptoms in an irritated or inflamed digestive tract.

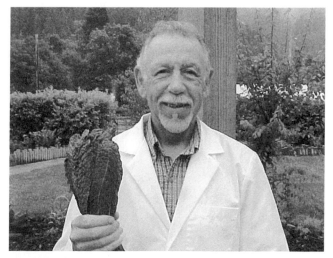

Dr. Paul Fieber

For many, the reflux of stomach content into the esophagus has more to do with inadequate secretions of stomach acid leading to the putrification of food and the accompanying symptoms of gas, bloating, reflux, and belching. Antacid therapy may provide temporary relief but does nothing to get to the cure.

In our study each participant was given 10 HCL capsules, which were enough to challenge 4 meals. We asked our group to challenge meals that were high in protein and a substantial complex meal. They started with 1 capsule with the first meal and if they had no mild burning or irritation they were to increase to 2 capsules with the next meal and continue until they had a reaction or reached a total of 4 capsules with no reaction at all. Out of the 27 participants, only two people had a reaction with 1 capsule and at that time they discontinued the study. The rest of our group all had some degree of hypochlorhydria and went on to participate in the study. The ages ranged from 17 to 80. All the participants were asked not to change any other part of their diet.

After 30 days of drinking one quart of green smoothie each day, we then completed another HCL challenge test to see what improvement occurred over the month. One person dropped out in the middle of the study due to nausea. Out of the other 24 participants we had 16 of the group who showed improvement in their production of HCL. **It was remarkable to me that 66.7% of the participants showed such vast improvement.** I did not expect to see this much progress in such a short period of time. The fiber content and nutrient value of the green smoothies made for an incredible success. All the participants also noted many other improvements in their health, some of which were dramatic changes. [*Please see the testimonials at the end of this book.*]

I would like to also give my own personal testimonial as my wife and I had been drinking the green smoothies about two months before the study was conducted. My blood pressure, pulse rate, and cholesterol readings all improved substantially. We lost all cravings for cooked food and the

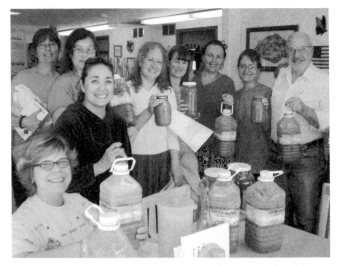

Raws'burg group (please see their personal testimonials in the back of the book)

green smoothies were both delicious and fulfilling. The most significant change for me concerned a small growth that had appeared on my nose. After one month on the green smoothies, the growth fell off and left a small hole where it once was. This proved to me the tremendous healing properties of the green smoothie.

I would like to personally thank Victoria for providing me the opportunity to contribute to such a remarkable study. I have met very few people in my life who have been as dedicated and have had such a passion for helping others. Thank you Victoria, you have changed our lives forever.

As Dr. Fieber mentioned, we were expecting some positive changes, but we didn't know they would be so significant in such a short period of time. Most experiments such as this one are usually planned for three to six months, but since the cost was out of our own pockets we did only what we could afford. The Roseburg Experiment demonstrated that regular consumption of green smoothies greatly benefits the health of people through improving the level of hydrochloric acid. Therefore the consumers of green smoothies should expect:

- to have better absorption of valuable nutrients;
- to lessen the possibility of infection and parasites;
- to heal allergies;
- to improve overall health.

Better absorption is in itself a great advantage. For example, better absorption of calcium may decrease the chances of osteoporosis, better absorption of iron may help to heal anemia; better absorption of B vitamins may protect against nerve disorders, and so on.

You may read personal testimonials of the Roseburg participants at the end of this book. As a result of regular consumption of the green smoothies for just one month, people named the following improvements: increase in energy, depression lifted and all suicidal thoughts gone, less blood sugar fluctuations, more regular bowel movements, dandruff healed, insomnia gone, asthma attacks stopped completely, none of usual "PMS" symptoms any more, fingernails became stronger, wanted less coffee, sex life improved, skin cleared up, and many more. It was interesting to see that most of the participants who wanted to lose weight lost anywhere from five to ten pounds, and a couple of people who wanted to gain weight, were able to gain one or two pounds.

The participants of the Roseburg Study were so excited about their results that some rumors got back to me that they were considering changing the name of their town to Raws'burg!

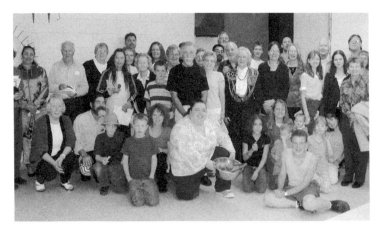

Raws'burg group with their families and friends.

The fact that all of the healing qualities of green smoothies were proven by practical experimentation makes this simple drink truly special. Please note that I am not trying to sell anything. I am hoping to inspire as many people as possible to incorporate green smoothies into their everyday lives.

From Roseburg to St. Petersburg

I am thrilled to let everyone know that a new, more detailed study similar to the Roseburg study has begun in Russia, at The Health Nutritional Center ROSTKI in St. Petersburg. For eight years, this center has been conducting various studies of the implications of chlorophyll on human health under the guidance of medical doctors, professors and scientists. The budget was approved for conducting a study of the effect of drinking green smoothies on the concentration of HCL in the stomach and on vitamin B-12 level.

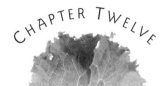

CHAPTER TWELVE

Greens Make the Body More Alkaline

$\int$ ometimes I feel that in our search for health, we have been going over the same ground for many decades. In the meantime, the most prevalent illness, cancer, is getting worse every year. Let us look at the statistics for the year 2005.[40]

- It is estimated 1,372,910 new cancer cases and 570,260 cancer deaths will occur; five-year survival rates have risen from 50 percent to 74 percent from the 1970s
- Lung cancer remains the biggest killer, estimated to claim the lives of 163,510 people
- About 232,090 men will be diagnosed with prostate cancer, killing 30,350
- Some 211,240 women will be diagnosed with breast cancer, killing 40,410

I have observed, both in Russia and in the United States, that mainstream medicine seems to have been focusing on the secondary causes of disease. To me that's like pushing a car that ran out of gas with your bare hands instead of putting gas in it, or comforting a hungry person instead of feeding them. So what is the main cause of disease?

Today we have an ocean of confusing information as well as articles in which different experts state many different reasons for illness. However, I think the main reason for illness was stated very clearly in 1931! Over 75 years ago Otto Warburg was awarded the Nobel prize for his discovery that cancer is caused by weakened cell respiration due to lack of oxygen at the cellular level. According to Warburg, damaged cell respiration causes fermentation, resulting in low pH (acidity) at the cellular level.

Dr. Warburg, in his Nobel Prize winning study, illustrated the environment of the cancer cell. A normal healthy cell undergoes an adverse change when it can no longer take in oxygen to convert glucose into energy. In the absence of oxygen, the cell reverts to a primal nutritional program to nourish itself by converting glucose through the process of fermentation. The lactic acid produced by fermentation lowers the cell pH (acid/alkaline balance) and destroys the ability of DNA and RNA to control cell division. The cancer cells then begin to multiply. The lactic acid simultaneously causes severe local pain as it destroys cell enzymes. Cancer appears as a rapidly growing external cell covering, with a core of dead cells.

Dr. Otto Warburg finished one of his most famous speeches with the following statement: "... *nobody today can say that one does not know what cancer and its prime cause is. On the contrary, **there is no disease whose prime cause is***

better known, *so that today ignorance is no longer an excuse that one cannot do more about prevention.*"[41]

Otto Warburg won the Nobel Prize for showing that cancer thrives in anaerobic (without oxygen), or acidic, conditions. In other words, the main cause for cancer is acidity of the human body. By the time I read his genius speech, he had been dead a long time. I wonder, if this discovery was so important that he received the Nobel Prize, why doesn't everyone know what pH is?

As soon as scientists discovered what healthy human blood pressure and temperature were supposed to be, devices were invented to measure them. Whenever I went to a doctor, my blood pressure and temperature were measured, but I don't ever remember a doctor measuring my pH. High blood pressure and fever, though not pleasant, do not cause cancer. The acidic condition of the blood does. This is what the internationally renowned scientist Dr. Warburg has proven. Therefore it seems vital to make pH information available at once to everyone.

It makes great sense to me that children should study the pH index of all foods at school and that all foods sold to the public should have their pH index printed on the content label together with calories and nutrients. For example, parmesan cheese should have a red warning label with a pH sign saying it is extremely acid forming, −34! While spinach may have a golden medal sign with a pH index +14, as an excellent, alkalizing food. The pH indexes have been measured in biochemical laboratories and cannot be guessed by just looking at foods. Some of the foods are surprisingly alkaline or acidic; for example, most people are amazed to learn that lemon is one of the most alkalizing fruits, while walnuts are slightly acidifying. I think it's important for the U.S. Department of Agriculture's food pyramid to reflect the pH of different foods as soon as possible. I imagine that many people's health could instantly be improved by their ability to consume alkalizing foods that are more beneficial for human health. You may find a complete list of pH values of different foods in the book *The pH Miracle* by Robert Young.

Fats as the main contributor to weight gain is a popular delusion among dieters. This misconception leads to massive confusion and explains **why so many overweight people are not succeeding in losing weight**. I am sure that many people would be shocked to find out that we may gain weight from eating, say, cheese, not only because it is rich in fat, but mostly due to its high acidic level. In response to high pH acid, the body creates fat cells to store the acid. For example, almonds have 70% fat, and pork has only 58%. However, pork has one of the highest acid values, −38, while almonds are alkaline forming, +3.[42] This is why it is so crucial to know, in addition to nutritional value, the pH index — to have it available and handy at every store, printed on each food label, showing its ability to alkalize the body. Knowing the pH indexes of various foods can help us balance our personal daily meal plans.

I remember how in 1965 my mother was in tears after reading an article in a Russian health magazine that stated that watermelons and cucumbers do not have any nutritional value. They were our family's most favorite foods. Forty years later, I am learning that cucumbers and watermelons are so alkalizing that they neutralize the acidifying effect of eating beef. I am glad that my parents continued to buy watermelons, despite "scientific" recommendations.

Many years ago, back in Russia, when I was studying to be a medical nurse, our professor told us that the cholesterol in our food did not contribute to the cholesterol level in our blood because it was our own liver that made cholesterol. Therefore, I was not surprised or disappointed by the diet high in fat and animal protein that my father was receiving while staying at the cardio center. After my dad's massive heart attack, they served him beefsteak with gravy and milk. Later, after reading a lot of books and articles about the importance of the proper pH balance in the body, I understood that the so-called "bad" cholesterol, lipoprotein (LDL) is made by our own liver in order to bind the toxins and deactivate the acidic waste that comes from certain foods, such as fats and animal protein. Unfortunately, I bought my first book on this topic, "Alkalize or Die"[43] two months after my father died from his second heart attack.

Food is not the only factor to affect our pH balance. Any stress can potentially leave an acidic residue in our body; conversely any activities that are calming and relaxing can make us more alkaline.

Factors that potentially make us more acid include hearing or saying harsh or bitter words, loud music and noise, being in a traffic jam, feeling jealousy or wanting revenge, hearing a baby crying, overworking and over-exercising, beginning or finishing school, going on vacation, watching scary or stressful movies, watching and listening to TV, talking on the phone for a long time, taking on a mortgage, paying bills and credit cards, etc.

Factors that potentially make us more alkaline are: giving or receiving a smile or a hug, laughter and jokes, classical or quiet music, seeing a puppy, hearing a compliment or blessing, receiving a soft massage, staying in a cozy and clean environment, being in nature, watching children laugh and play, walking and sleeping under the stars and moonlight, working in the garden, observing flowers, singing or playing a musical instrument, sincere friendly conversation, and many others.

I find it helpful to observe my inner body's reaction to different events around me, and if I notice unwanted feeling of inner stress, I try to make changes not only to my diet but to my whole way of living.

Being uneducated about pH balance breeds a lot of confusion among people who are looking for healthy diets. They try many different things very often without positive results. For example, in my own experience, I have been eating only raw food for many years. While this was a vast improvement over my previous diet, I did not reach the optimal results I desired until I began to eat more greens. I read several books and articles on this subject and bought litmus paper with which to measure my pH. However, every time I measured my saliva or urine, it was almost always acid. So I got even more confused and stopped measuring. I was convinced that my diet was the best it could be because what could be better than a raw food diet? I never understood the importance of keeping the alkaline balance of my body.

Since I started drinking green smoothies, I decided to check my pH balance once again. I tested both my saliva and urine and was surprised to see that my litmus paper was now the stable green color of alkalinity!

As soon as I clearly noticed the tight connection between the food that we intake and our pH balance, I purchased for my family plenty of pH measurement tape and placed it in the bathrooms and kitchens, available at any time, so we could check our pH balance every day and rest assured that our health is out of danger. After staying so many years on a 100% raw diet, I have come to the conclusion that it is **impossible to maintain a good alkaline pH balance without consuming large quantities of dark leafy greens**, approximately two bunches or one to two pounds every day. Some people try to keep a normal pH balance by taking supplements containing dried greens. While this is certainly better than eating only French fries, I strongly believe that to consume fresh greens is thousands of times better because supplements are processed food and their nutritional content is altered, as a result of which some qualities of the nutrients disappear so that the value of the nutrients changes greatly. Also, when consumed in forms of capsules and tablets, they enter our body in huge, concentrated doses, and any additional nutrients create extra work for the elimination system.

For this reason, out of all the choices that we have in consuming greens, the green smoothie is a winner because it is a complete food, it is fresh, and it takes less than a minute to prepare.

CHAPTER THIRTEEN

Healthy Soil is More Valuable than Gold

"We are the dust of the Earth."
DR. BERNARD JENSEN

When I read my first book on permaculture, (which is a natural way of gardening), I unexpectedly learned such stunning facts about soil that I have radically changed many of my habits. In addition to composting, recycling, and buying only organic food, I now have a small permaculture garden of my own. Most importantly, I have developed a deep respect for all soils.

During the hundreds of millions of years that plants have been living on our planet, they have become amazingly self-sufficient. In addition to obtaining a useful relationship with the sun, plants have learned to "grow" their own soil! When plants die, it may look to us like they just fall on the ground and rot, getting eaten by multitudes of bugs and worms. However, researchers were shocked to discover that dead plants get consumed only by particular bacteria and fungi.[44] Plants "know" how to attract to their own rotting only those

microorganisms and earthworms, that will produce beneficial minerals for the soil where the plants' siblings will grow.
One way plants attract particular microorganisms into their
soil is by concentrating more sugars in their roots. Thus
roots, like carrots and potatoes, are always much sweeter
than the rest of the plant. Plants and microorganisms develop a symbiotic relation, beneficial to both plant and
microbe.[45] Just like humans with our farm animals, plants
"breed" certain microorganisms and specific kinds of fungi
that produce the humus (organic matter) that is rich in the
most useful minerals for these plants. Apparently, the quality of the soil is critically important, not only as a source of
water and minerals for plants, but essentially vital for their
very survival. That is why plants must never be researched
separately from the soil they grow in.

If we care which nutrients we receive from plants, we
absolutely cannot ignore the quality of nutrients plants receive
from the soil because **we literally consume minerals from the
soil through plants.** The quality of the soil in which plants
grow has an immense influence on the health of the people
and animals who eat plants. The following example with
pure-bred horses clearly demonstrates the impact soil can
have on people and animals: "Within a few generations, the
originally giant dappled Percheron draft horses, developed on
the soils of a French district south of Normandy, had dwindled to the size of Cossack horses, though their bloodlines
had been kept pure by the Soviets and their confirmation
remained the same, though miniaturized."[46] This case reveals
that the soils plants grow in are as important to our health as
plants themselves, if not more so! In other words, as odd as it

sounds, **our well-being depends on the quality of the land in which our food grows** because the original source of nutrients for humans comes from soils, not plants.

The main difference between organic and conventional gardening is that "Conventional agriculture attempts to feed the plants while the organic method nourishes the microorganisms in soil."[47] In simple words, conventional farmers ignore the microorganisms in the soil and aim their efforts at supplying potassium, nitrogen and other chemicals for the sake of plants, while organic gardeners take care of feeding the living things in the soil, which provide harmoniously balanced nutrients to the plants. Just as humans cannot live on chemicals instead of food, microorganisms in the soil cannot survive when fed artificial fertilizers. **When all microorganisms get destroyed with chemicals, the soil turns to dust.** No plants can grow in dust, no matter how rich in various chemicals this dust is.

Through the plants we eat, we receive essential nutrients that were created by microorganisms in the soil. The more organic mater or humus is in the soil, the more nutritious is the food grown on this soil.

In the following table please see the astonishing differences in nutritional content between organically and conventionally grown produce.[48] Check out, for example, the iron content in tomatoes and spinach. Also make note of the fact that there is almost no cobalt in conventionally grown produce. Since cobalt serves as the base for the B-12 vitamin (Cobalamin) I wonder if consuming predominately conventionally grown veggies could contribute to B-12 deficiencies.

Plants seem to be much better "farmers" than we are. As a

Organic Produce vs. Conventional Produce

Vegetable	Total Mineral Ash	Phosphorous	Calcium	Magnesium	Potassium	Sodium
	Percentage of dry weight			Millequivalents per 100 grams dry weight		
Snap Beans						
Organic	10.45	0.36	40.5	60.0	99.7	8.6
Commercial	4.04	0.22	15.5	14.8	29.1	0.9
Cabbage						
Organic	10.38	0.38	60.0	43.6	148.3	20.4
Commercial	6.12	0.18	17.5	13.6	33.7	0.8
Lettuce						
Organic	24.48	0.43	71.0	49.3	176.5	12.2
Commercial	7.01	0.22	16.0	13.1	53.7	0.0
Tomatoes						
Organic	14.20	0.35	23.0	59.2	148.3	6.5
Commercial	6.07	0.16	4.5	4.5	58.8	0.0
Spinach						
Organic	28.56	0.52	96.0	203.9	237.0	69.5
Commercial	12.38	0.27	47.5	46.9	84.6	0.0

result of their clever "gardening" for millions of years, we humans have inherited many feet of beautiful fruitful topsoil all around the globe with zillions of happy microorganisms thriving in it. In their best-selling book, Secrets of the Soil, Peter Tompkins and Christopher Bird state that, "The combined weight of all the microbial cells on earth is twenty-five times that of its animal life; every acre of well-cultivated land contains up to a half a ton of thriving microorganisms, and a ton of earthworms which can daily excrete a ton of humic castings."[49]

As a result of our human "highly technological" garden-

	Trace amounts parts per million dry matter			
Boron	Manganese	Iron	Copper	Cobalt
73.0	60.0	227.0	69.0	0.26
10.0	2.0	10.0	3.0	0.00
42.0	13.0	94.0	48.0	0.15
7.0	2.0	20.0	0.4	0.00
37.0	169.0	516.0	60.0	0.19
6.0	1.0	9.0	3.0	0.00
36.0	68.0	1938.0	53.0	0.63
3.0	1.0	1.0	0.0	0.00
88.0	117.0	1584.0	32.0	0.25
12.0	1.0	49.0	0.3	0.20

ing, most of the soil of agricultural farms in the USA contains less than 2% of organic matter, while originally, before the era of chemistry, it was 60–100%. According to David Blume, an ecological biologist, permaculture teacher and expert, "Most Class I commercial agricultural soil is lucky to hit 2% organic matter — the dividing line between a living and dead soil."[50] By applying permaculture gardening techniques to a field of extremely depleted soil, which consisted of cement-hard adobe clay, David Blume was able to bring the organic matter to the 25% level within a couple of years.

From this field he harvested the crops "8 times what the USDA claims are possible per square foot."[51]

We cannot successfully feed soils with chemicals because "biology does not equal chemistry."[52] In other words, chemical fertilizers are missing live enzymes which contribute to the most unique qualities of all soils. According to the abundance of research done in different countries, **soil enzymes can transform one element into another** if such "biological transmutation" would benefit the plants that grow in this soil. Take a look at the following quotes from numerous studies and see for yourself.

Professor Rene Furon, of the Faculty of Sciences at Paris University states, "It can no longer be denied that **nature makes magnesium out of calcium** (in some cases the reverse takes place); that **potassium can come from sodium**."[53]

Komaki, head of a biological research laboratory at the Matsushita Electric Company in Japan states, "Various microorganisms, including certain bacteria and two species each of molds and yeasts, were capable of transmuting **sodium into potassium**."[54]

Professor P. A. Korolkov in Russia states, ". . . **silicon can be converted to aluminum** . . . we are being subjected to a radical revision, not of minutiae, but of the basic status of an inherited natural science. The time has come to recognize that **any chemical element can turn into another**, under natural conditions."[55]

These are the solid facts from which we can conclude that chemical fertilizers could never enrich the living soil but could only damage or even destroy it with the most devastating consequences for plants, animals, and people.

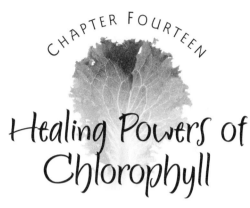

CHAPTER FOURTEEN

Healing Powers of Chlorophyll

*"The moment one gives close attention to anything,
even a blade of grass, it becomes a mysterious, awesome,
indescribably magnificent world in itself."*
HENRY MILLER

The longer I live my life, the more I acquire admiration for nature. When hiking in the morning, if I run into a deer, squirrel, or any other creature, I freeze and "absorb them with my eyes" so zealously as if nothing else matters for me. I sense a great mystery in animals, flowers, trees, and especially in the sun. When I look at the sun, I appreciate that the sunshine is free and equally available for everyone.

Many people enjoy the sun. We all feel better and look healthier if we regularly spend time in the sun. We attempt to get as much sunlight as possible. Our bathing suits have become reduced to the very minimum as we are trying to immerse our bodies in the precious sunshine. However, not many people are aware of the sunlight's liquefied form, chlorophyll.

Chlorophyll is as important as sunlight! No life is possible without sunshine and no life is possible without chlorophyll. Chlorophyll is liquefied sun energy. Consuming as much chlorophyll as possible is exactly like bathing our inner organs in sunshine. The molecule of chlorophyll is remarkably similar to the molecule of heme, human blood.[56] Chlorophyll takes care of our body like a most caring and loving mother. It heals and cleanses all our organs and even destroys many of our internal enemies, like pathogenic bacteria, fungus, cancer cells,[57] and many others.

To experience optimal health we need to have 80–85% of "good" bacteria in our intestines. Friendly bacteria manufacture many essential nutrients for our body, including vitamin K, B-vitamins, numerous helpful enzymes and other vital substances. Such "good" or **aerobic bacteria** thrive in the presence of oxygen and require it for their continued growth and existence. That is why if we do not have enough oxygen in the cells of our body, "bad" bacteria take over and begin to thrive, causing an extreme amount of infections and disease. These pathogenic bacteria are **anaerobic**, and cannot tolerate gaseous oxygen. Taking care of our intestinal flora is vitally important! "Good" bacteria could be easily destroyed with countless factors, like antibiotics, poor diet, overeating, stress, etc. In this case we could have 80–90% of "bad" bacteria filling our body with toxic acidic waste. I believe that the dominance of anaerobic bacteria in our intestines is the prime cause of all disease.

Since ancient times chlorophyll has served as a miraculous healer. Chlorophyll carries significant amounts of oxygen with it and thus plays a critical role in supporting the aerobic bacteria. Therefore, the more chlorophyll we consume, the better our intestinal flora and overall health will be. Considering that greens are a major source of chlorophyll, **it is difficult to find a better way of consuming chlorophyll than drinking green smoothies.**

Chlorophyll has been proven helpful in preventing and healing many forms of cancer[58] and arteriosclerosis.[59] Abundant scientific research shows that there are hardly any illnesses that could not be helped by chlorophyll. In order to describe all remedial qualities of chlorophyll I would have to write a whole separate volume. So I have listed only some of the many healing properties of this amazing substance.

Chlorophyll
- ❀ Builds a high blood count
- ❀ Helps prevent cancer
- ❀ Provides iron to organs
- ❀ Makes body more alkaline
- ❀ Counteracts toxins eaten
- ❀ Improves anemic conditions
- ❀ Cleans and deodorizes bowel tissues
- ❀ Helps purify the liver
- ❀ Aids hepatitis improvement
- ❀ Regulates menstruation
- ❀ Aids hemophilia condition
- ❀ Improves milk production
- ❀ Helps sores heal faster
- ❀ Eliminates body odors
- ❀ Resists bacteria in wounds
- ❀ Cleans tooth and gum structure in pyorrhea
- ❀ Eliminates bad breath

- Relieves sore throat
- Makes an excellent oral surgery gargle
- Benefits inflamed tonsils
- Soothes ulcer tissues
- Soothes painful hemorrhoids and piles
- Aids catarrhal discharges
- Revitalizes vascular system in the legs
- Improves varicose veins
- Reduces pain caused by inflammation
- Improves vision

The most important goal of all life forms on our planet is a continuation of their life. What do we humans need to survive? Besides air and water, our primary need is food. We get our food from plants and animals. Where do plants get their food? Plants obtain their food from the soil and directly from the sun! **Only plants "know" how to convert sunlight into carbohydrates**. That is how plants grow. They make carbohydrates out of sunlight, from carbohydrates plants build new stems, roots and bark, and most importantly, they build new leaves because leaves can make more carbohydrates. This is why the mass of leaves is always superior in size in relation to the rest of the plant. Since the greens are always trying to increase absorption of chlorophyll, they continuously keep growing and, as a result, we have to constantly trim the bushes and cut the grass around our homes; otherwise the greens will keep growing without stopping until they take over the entire space, leaving no room for us.

Plants' lives depend on sunshine and our life depends on plants. Even when people eat animals they eat them for the sake of the nutrients that the animal received earlier through consuming plants. That is why humans almost never eat carnivorous animals, but only the ones that eat plants. Ancient Palestine teachings, Islam, and various other religions prohibit the eating of carnivorous animals like lions, tigers, leopards, fox, eagles, pelicans, etc. My grandmother recalled that during the war, her hungry relatives tried eating the meat of carnivorous animals and birds and all became violently sick. At the same time, no living creatures, even carnivores, could survive without consuming some greens. We all notice how dogs and cats occasionally eat green grass.

With high oxygen content in chlorophyll and high mineral content in green plants, greens are the most alkalizing food that exists on our planet. By including green smoothies into our diet we can keep our bodies alkaline and healthy.

Another great way to get chlorophyll and nutrients from greens is drinking wheatgrass juice. This highly nourishing drink was invented by Dr. Ann Wigmore and is becoming more and more popular all the time. Wheatgrass juice consists of 70% chlorophyll and contains 92 different minerals out of 102 possible, beta carotene and the B vitamins, plus C, E, H and K, 19 amino acids and beneficial enzymes. All of these properties make wheatgrass an extraordinary health builder.

However, the strong nutritional density of wheatgrass juice makes it hard to drink for many people. Many would like to regularly consume it but cannot do so because of nauseous reactions sometimes caused from the smell alone. I also tried many times to start drinking wheatgrass and could not keep it down even after learning the special "wheatgrass dance," saying a special prayer, clipping my nose, and other tricks.

After drinking green smoothies regularly for one year, I was offered a shot of wheatgrass and unexpectedly, loved it! Now, for the first time in my life I am able to comfortably drink 4, 6, 8 or more ounces of wheatgrass each day. I was so amazed and pleased that for a while I continued to visit our local Ashland Co-op to drink wheatgrass, paying $10–$15 at a time just for this drink. I heard the girls that work at the juice bar telling each other that they never saw anybody drinking so much of it so easily. None of them could drink any wheatgrass at all! Now I don't consume it daily, but if I have a chance I always go for it. I think that this dramatic change in my body's acceptance of wheatgrass has to do with my improved level of stomach acid.

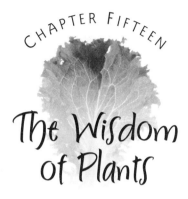

CHAPTER FIFTEEN

The Wisdom of Plants

We have already discussed the sophisticated relationship plants have with soil and sunshine. Apparently, millions of years of co-existence on the same planet have resulted in plants, people, and animals developing a strong symbiotic connection. Plants do not mind if people and animals eat their fruits because such practice benefits the plant by spreading its seeds for future generations. In fact plants are "interested" in someone eating their fruit, but only when it is ripe. As I stated before, the goal of all plants is the continuation of their species and providing adequate living conditions for them. That is why nearly nearly all the fruits in the world have a round shape, so that it could roll away and start a new life. For the very same reason plants have learned to make their fruit colorful, palatable, and nutritious to ensure that its consumers not only eat one fruit but continue to return for more. This strategy works very well and all fruit gets eaten. Have you ever noticed how thoroughly birds "clean" cherry trees or how squirrels keep working on an oak tree until there are no more acorns left? What happens next? The "eaters" digest their food and have bowel movements far away from the mother plant and the seeds are covered with nice "organic fertilizer." The seeds get a perfect start. Inside the fruit, the seeds are wisely protected from being digested with hardy shells and inhibitors. Note that the plant keeps its fruit extremely un-tasteful, colorless, and without attractive fragrance all the way until the seeds are ripe, so that nobody wastes them before the seeds have matured.

The following example illustrates how much the continuation of their species means to plants. In a recent study in Russia, biologists discovered that "When a tree is foreseeing its death, the tree gathers its entire energy and deposits this energy into producing seeds for the very last time. For example, the oak tree broken by the storm or the cedar tree with its bark removed from its trunk, in a farewell effort before they die forever, give their record crops of acorns or nuts."[60]

In contrast with the previous example, when a plant is genetically altered, it does not produce seeds on purpose. Such a plant makes itself infertile to prevent future unhealthy generations. Seedless watermelons are usually odorless and tasteless, because an upset plant has no motivation to make its fruits sweet, fragrant, or attractive in any other way. I am sure that it is not healthy to eat seedless plants, because their entire chemistry, electromagnetic charge, and who knows what else has been altered. In my own life, I prefer to pay double for an organic seeded watermelon or tomato.

Do plants "want" us to eat their trunk and roots? Nope.

That is why the roots are hidden in the ground. The roots are for the microorganisms in the soil, as we described in the previous chapter. The trunk is purposely covered with hard and bitter bark. And what about the greens? Again, plants demonstrate their perfect ability to develop symbiosis with different creatures. Plants "allow" humans and animals to eat all of their fruits, but only part of their leaves, because plants need to have leaves for their own use — which is manufacturing chlorophyll. However, plants depend on moving creatures for many different reasons, like pollination, fertilizing the soil, and hanging around to help eat the ripe fruit. For this reason, plants accumulate a lot of highly nutritious elements in their leaves, but mix these nourishing ingredients with either bitterness or very small amounts of alkaloids (poisons). That is how animals are forced to rotate their menu and that is why all wild animals are browsers. They eat a small amount of one thing, then move on to many other plants during the course of the day. The body is capable of detoxifying small amounts of a great many things. Chimpanzees also rotate the green plants they eat. They go through approximately 117 different plants in one year.[61] We humans need to learn to alternate our variety of greens as much as possible instead of eating only iceberg lettuce, spinach and romaine. I was able to locate only about 40 types of various greens, including edible weeds, that are available in my state of Oregon. I hope that our farmers will learn to grow a larger variety of green leafy vegetables to increase our green sources. The following is a list of greens that my family has been rotating in our diet during the last year.

Greens
Arugula
Asparagus
Beet greens (tops)
Bok choy
Broccoli
Carrot tops
Celery
Chard
Collard greens
Edible Flowers
Endive
Escarole
Frisee
Kale (3 types)
Mizuna
Mustard greens
Radicchio
Radish tops
Romaine lettuce, green
  and red leaf (no Iceberg
  or light colored leaf)
Spinach

Weeds
Chickweed
Clover
Dandelion (greens
  & Flowers)
Lambsquarters
Malva
Miner's lettuce
Plantain
Purslane
Stinging Nettles

Herbs
Aloe Vera
Baby Dill
Basil
Cilantro
Fennel
Mint
Parsley (2 types)
Peppermint leaves
Spearmint

Sprouts
Alfalfa
Broccoli
Clover
Fenugreek
Radish
Sunflower

Wild edibles often contain more vitamins and minerals than commercially marketed plants. Weeds have not been "spoiled" with farmers' care in contrast to the "good" plants of the garden. In order to survive in spite of constant weeding, pulling, and spraying, weeds had to develop strong survival properties. For example, in order to stay alive without being watered, most weeds have developed unbelievably long roots. Alfalfa's roots grow up to 20 feet long reaching for the most fertile layers of the soil. As a result, all wild plants possess more nutrients than commercially grown plants. I feel so silly now when I remember how I used to always pull out the "nasty" lambsquarters from my garden to let my "precious" iceberg lettuce grow.

While there are countless benefits associated with eating wild foods, there are also some risks. It is a good idea to first learn how to positively identify the edible plants. I urge you to **take caution when harvesting wild foods**. Eating wild edibles is fun, healthful, and safe when done properly. Please take the time to educate yourself and your loved ones. If you are ever in doubt about whether a plant is edible or not, please, please don't eat it!

The best way to learn which weeds are edible is to sign up for an herb walk with an experienced guide in your local area. This way you can learn to recognize particular edible plants by actually touching, smelling, and tasting them so that you can gather your "wild produce" on your own. Also, there are lots of articles and photos of edible weeds on the internet. You may also find many books that help identify edible plants in your area.

For variety, we include several kinds of sprouts in our diet, but never more than a handful and only one or two times a week. Approximately from the third to the sixth day of their life, sprouts contain higher levels of alkaloids, as a means of protection from animals nipping them off and killing them.[62] That doesn't mean that sprouts are poisonous or dangerous, but only that we cannot live on sprouts alone. Most sprouts are rich in B-vitamins and have a hundred times more nutrients than a fully developed plant because sprouts need more nutrition for their fast growing period.

Once in a while I read in the news or receive an e-mail

about kale or spinach or parsley or any other green having a toxic ingredient and therefore being dangerous for human consumption. This is all true but not to a degree as to exclude any particular green from our diet. Let us learn to increase the variety of greens in our diet and to constantly rotate them for better nutritional results.

There are several other ways in which plants protect themselves from being destroyed. Some plants have thorns instead of alkaloids and one type of acacia tree in Africa is inhabited by colonies of very aggressive ants with a painful sting.

Thorny plants, like cactuses and stinging nettles, do not contain any alkaloids which makes them a valuable addition to our diet. Of course, we need to first figure out how to eat them. I have often successfully added stinging nettles to my green smoothies.

Cereal grasses contain very little or no alkaloids because they attempt to attract deer, wild horses, goats, and other animals to the meadows in order to collect fertilizer from these animals. Grasses' leaf texture evolved to be coarse and hard to digest, thus forcing animals to stay in the meadows all day long chewing.

When I think about all these little tricks plants have developed for their survival, I feel an immense respect and admiration for nature. Our symbiosis with plants has developed over a course of millions of years, but we could ruin it in just a matter of decades. I believe that we still can repair our relationship with nature. Returning back to our original diet is one necessary step towards this goal.

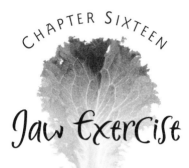

CHAPTER SIXTEEN

Jaw Exercise

I realized that by consuming most of my food in a blended form, I had almost completely eliminated chewing, which I knew was an important part of the digestive process. I decided to create some exercises for my jaws and eventually came up with a jaw exerciser; a simple device that I started carrying around with me to practice jaw workouts when I had a chance.

At first I was amazed how weak my jaws were. They would get numb after as few as five movements. I kept progressing very quickly and by the end of the second day of practicing I was able to perform 20–30 movements at once.

I have to admit that moving my jaws against the resisting force of the exerciser is pleasant to such a degree that I actually enjoy it. I realize how much my jaws have longed for this kind of movement all these years. In addition to this pleasant sensation, I have noticed that my teeth have become whiter and a lot stronger. My gums became healthier. I also noticed that performing a little workout in my mouth right before eating improved my digestion.

I did some research and found out that bone tissue that forms our skeleton is a truly remarkable material. It is constantly modeling and remodeling itself. This process of continuous bone regeneration reminds me of our road service that is constantly performing construction on highways, taking old cracked pavement off, and laying down new strong smooth asphalt instead. Furthermore, the roads that are used most heavily get more attention and better concrete, while the roads that are rarely used stay overlooked and eroded.

In 1892 a German doctor, J. Wolff, discovered that, "Mechanical forces have a major influence on the bone modeling and remodeling processes in both cortical and trabecular bone, since their effects on bone morphology are obvious . . . The mechanical forces are sensed in the bone, and all of these mechanical forces are translated to structural adaptation of the internal tissue architecture."[63] Dr. Wolff has explained that our bones can strengthen or weaken in response to the forces applied to them. In other words, when we load our bones with work, as a response to such a workout, our bones result in higher bone mineral density, and thus become stronger. A recent medical study in Manchester, UK, demonstrated that, "The playing arm of adult tennis players has up to 40% more bone mass than the non-playing arm."[64] On the contrary, if we do not exercise, our bones detrain and lose strength from inactivity. For example, astronauts in space lose some of their bone mass due to an absence of gravity. In conclusion, to strengthen our bones we need to exercise. No pills, food, or supplements can substitute for exercise to make our bones stronger.

Many people have problems both with the narrowing of their jaws and thinning of the jawbone. "It's a major problem in dentistry," said Ichiro Nishimura, associate professor of restorative dentistry at Harvard School of Dental Medicine. "The thin jaws can be easily fractured. Also, placing dentures is very difficult, since there's no supporting structure." One way to solve these problems would be to get the jawbone to grow new supporting bone. But this solution has the ring of a fantasy, something for a future age.[65]

Dr. Weston Price[66] was deeply concerned with the fast growing number of increasingly deformed dental arches, crooked teeth, and cavities. In 1939 he wrote about a profound degeneration of health in so-called civilized nations. That was almost 100 years ago. In his research, Price demonstrated the connection between the development of jaw deformities and eating processed foods. I would like to emphasize that raw, natural, unprocessed food requires a lot of chewing, while most processed foods are too soft and do not need any work on behalf of jaw muscles. For example, compare soft wonder bread, baked potato or oatmeal (which hardly need chewing at all), to some tough plants such as, celery stalks, hard-shelled nuts or fibrous roots that require vigorous masticating. The absence of a workout for the muscles of our jaws is probably one of the major factors contributing to the development of weak, narrow, degenerative jaws.

I am currently perfecting my own jaw exerciser, and am planning to start commerically distributing it in 2006. My dentist told me that there are millions of Americans who suffer from severe jaw deformity. Especially many young people and children. He said that they usually have to go through a very painful surgery that gives them only temporarily relief. I hope that some dentists will consider including my jaw exercise program into their prevention recommendations.

CHAPTER SEVENTEEN

A Tribute to Dr. Ann

I truly admire Dr. Ann Wigmore. Whenever I order a shot of wheatgrass, I feel like I personally know Dr. Ann. Wheatgrass juice makes me healthier. I owe the opportunity of drinking it at my local co-op to Dr. Ann. Thanks to her, people in the whole world can drink wheatgrass juice and enjoy its countless healing benefits. I find it amazing how Ann Wigmore is continuing to touch our lives many years after she has passed away, even though many of us have never met her, or even heard her name.

Not only did Dr. Ann discover and thoroughly research the great healing properties of wheatgrass, but she also developed and thoroughly described the process of growing wheatgrass in trays at home or any location. She came up with an inexpensive wheatgrass juicer to make this elixir of life available to everyone.

I appreciate many of Dr. Ann's inventions which we all conveniently utilize in our everyday lives while thinking that they have existed forever. Who remembers today that raw gourmet food began with Dr. Ann's "seed cheese" and "raw soup" recipes. She invented for us "nut milks" and dehydrated crackers, "almond loaf" and "live" candy.

Dr. Ann introduced a variety of sprouts into our lives. She also came up with a sprouting bag. Whenever my family travels, we always pack sprouting seeds to guarantee a fresh supply of greens. Dr. Ann called sprouts Living Foods. It is hard to imagine that these words didn't exist some time ago.

Dr. Ann discovered the many healing benefits of blending foods, especially greens. Dr Ann Wigmore lived the last several years of her life **almost completely on blended foods, a large part of which consisted of greens.** She noticed that blended foods were assimilated more easily. For instance, she would say about fruit, "If I have an apple, I will blend it instead of munch it, because I don't want to waste its energy or mine." She observed that eating blended food gave her superior health and cut her hours of sleep down to two hours per night.[67]

Before Dr. Ann, people utilized blenders for "insignificant" purposes like whipping eggs and making cocktails. Today, we cannot imagine a raw food kitchen without a powerful blender.

Dr. Ann Wigmore clearly saw the tight connection between organic soil and human health, and she began promoting organic gardening and composting in the sixties when most people were just beginning to embrace chemical fertilizers as the future of agriculture.

I see Ann Wigmore's uniqueness in her ability to pay attention to a wide spectrum of events, to explore living on this planet as one whole process, and to apply her expertise to many different aspects of life. She didn't choose to be a specialist in just one narrow field as many others have done. She dared to form her personal opinion about everything she encountered, be it blood analysis, colonic irrigations, fasting, food composition, bacteria, gardening, or drinking water. Due to her all-inclusive vision, she was able to create a healing system that has helped thousands of people.

Dr. Ann was known to work vigorously and productively. She invented new ideas daily. She kept herself in notably excellent shape, always running, never walking, sustaining herself on just two hours of sleep per day. At the ripe age of 82, Dr. Ann didn't have a single gray hair. This fact was so unbelievable that her students asked her permission to study her hair in a lab to see if it was dyed. The test proved that it was her natural color.

In addition to her profound research in the field of human health, Dr. Ann was an animal rights activist, she fought against the fluoridation and chlorination of drinking water, against chemical pollution, and many other things.

The latest discoveries in science prove Dr. Ann was right in the majority of her predictions and recommendations. I believe the day will come when medical students will study Ann Wigmore's books as they study Hippocrates today.

Dr. Ann is well recognized all around the world. In my

travels I continue to encounter people who ask me if I have heard of Dr. Ann Wigmore. This inquiry is usually followed by an exciting story about another human life saved by Dr. Ann's teachings. I doubt it is possible to calculate just how many lives this brilliant woman has saved. She herself was one of the healthiest people on the planet in the 20th century. Dr. Ann was living her talk and practicing in her own life everything that she was teaching. Most of all, however, people who met her in person remember her for her benevolent loving spirit.

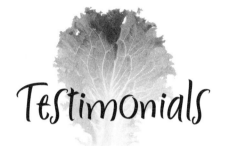

Testimonials

From Beef and Pork to Green Smoothie

This testimony goes out to all the "big fellows" out there. I was the guy who when given an option of beef or pork in my burrito said both and add some extra cheese while you're at it. I am the guy who was offended at the mention of it costing extra money for extra toppings. The very sight of my obvious excitement at an all-you-can-eat buffet caused the managers to quiver with fear. I was the guy who was shocked when asked if I would like salad with my steak. Salad? Can you imagine? No, send me some wings instead. I was the one who honestly believed that Rocky Road was not just an ice cream but, for the brave, a way of life. I loved this stuff and it was killing me.

I was grossly overweight and actually ashamed of myself. That's when my wife started researching about raw foods. One of her friends mentioned about the green smoothies. It was a bit thick but cleverly delicious. Each new dinner creation that my wife presented to me was both refreshing and pleasing to the eye. Don't get me wrong I wasn't instantly hooked, but after choosing to put my health first, I actually started to like it.

I have been drinking green smoothies a little more than three weeks now and I feel more alive than ever. Just the other morning I woke up before my alarm clock! That has happened a few times in a row now. I have never been a morning person and now I wake up with so much energy. It was almost scary to be so alert, but a welcome change. The most exciting thing is that now I crave the good stuff. The greener the better! I have lost a lot of weight. I really don't know how much but **I have gone down from a size 48 pants to now a 42 (almost 40) and I'm not done yet!** This is all still new for me, but I have felt the difference and I am not going back. Now, I have the energy and desire to exercise. I know the weight will keep coming off. The food is not only delicious but for all you super-sizers it's also surprisingly satisfying. So, to you my friend I say, "Jump in." Start living. This is real; this is good; this is right. Some people might say that I am extreme but I choose to say that I am RAW. A big shout-out to Victoria for teaching us how to eat healthy and to drink those delicious green smoothies. More Please! :)   — Mr. R.R.V.

Green Smoothie Helps to Prepare for a Marathon.

I've been a raw-fooder for over a year and a half now, and over the past few months, have given green smoothies a large role in my diet. I drink at least one almost every day. I'm currently training for my first marathon. Prior to this training, the furthest I had ever run was about three and a half miles. I had not been able to run further, because I always seemed to injure one of my knees, meaning I would have to stop running for weeks until it felt better. I also felt as though I could not possibly push myself to run farther. I'm happy to report that I am now up to 14 miles (which means I am a half-marathoner!) and not only have I not injured myself, but I also have not been the least bit sore the day after a run — even after running 8, 10, 12, and 14 miles! The other participants in my training group often complain of soreness, and I have been recovering very well. Sometimes I am a bit sore immediately following a run, but I always feel great the next day!

I notice that I have a lot of energy for a workout if I drink a green smoothie as a pre-workout meal. My favorite for a pre-workout meal is banana (or mango) with celery. This provides me with the sugars and electrolytes I need for the long runs in the summer heat.   — *B. E. from Chicago*

Wheelchair for sale!

Three months ago I counted my life as pretty much over. To me living was a slow dying and dying was the final end to my suffering. I am twenty-five and was in a wheelchair. I couldn't walk the ten feet from my bedroom to the couch in the living room without panting for air and feeling the spasms in my back start to take hold. I had been this way for over six months and I lost every hope of every being able to walk on my own again. I was beyond miserable; I was more than two hundred pounds overweight. To make matters worse, I also had advanced sleep apnea; it was so bad that I could not even use the C-PAP machine that most sufferers use because even at full power it did not provide me enough air to allow me to breathe at night. I never made it to REM sleep at all and most nights frequently woke up two to three times from lack of oxygen. I was beyond conventional help. Because of my poor sleep, I was exhausted all day long and I would literally fall asleep every five to ten minutes no matter what I was doing, or where I was. So my life became brief moments of being awake in pain and struggling to function as best I could before I fell asleep again. I was depressed all the time and cried on a daily basis, usually for nothing.

Then a month ago my aunt and uncle who are into raw foods invited me to come to Oregon and stay with them for a while and try raw foods to see if they could improve my health at all. I figured that I would give it a try — since nothing else had worked — and I was sure that the way I was living and by the severity of my health I would never see my thirtieth birthday. On my first day I decided to try and walk and within less than five minutes I was in tears. My back just wouldn't let me move. That day I went 100% raw and I started drinking Green Smoothies. I pushed myself every day to walk a little further. By the end of the first week I was able to walk the thirty feet to the barn, I could stay awake for hours and I even felt like I was starting to lose weight! It has been over two weeks now and I am still 100% raw. I have lost twenty-five pounds, I can stay awake for the whole day, and yesterday I even hiked, yes, hiked a quarter mile hill that is on the farm. I couldn't believe it! When I reached the top I sat down and cried, not because I was in pain, but because I walked! That is the farthest I have walked in over a year, and it's just the beginning! My whole attitude has changed too, I am no longer depressed, I have a positive outlook now. I feel like a new person inside and out. I know that I have been given a second chance to live and that raw foods saved my life. I will never go back to eating and living the way I was before. Who would want to trade this miracle of life and health for a few moments of food? Definitely not me. I think about all I have accomplished in two short weeks and I know that in the future I can do anything because I am alive now, and I have strength and energy. I would totally urge everyone to give raw foods a chance to help them improve the quality of their health and lives. I want everyone to feel as wonderful as I do.   —*J. S., Sacramento, CA*

Green Smoothies Help Normalize B-12 Level

I was allergic to all foods to such a degree that I could not sleep. I frequently called emergency and in one month I was hospitalized five times. I was diagnosed with chronic fatigue syndrome and Hypothyroidism in 1989. I felt confusion and muscle pain for five years, suffered allergies and candida then was hospitalized once. I couldn't work physically or dance. I wanted to die. I was given high doses of Xanax antibiotics for a hiatal hernia that did not help me at all and gave me heart palpitations (murmurs). At this point I became a vegan/vegetarian, which only made a slight improvement. Then I went on a raw food diet and started to feel a lot better right away. However my cholesterol was still high at 200. I was 90% Raw for about seven years. Most of my symptoms were gone except my B-12 was low. My doctor put me on B-12 shots and supplements.

Five months ago I added green smoothies to my diet and my health dramatically improved. I usually drink one quart a day. I like Lambsquarters or Kale as a base with parsley, pear, mango and apple. Sometimes I add papaya and soaked chia seeds. After four months my cholesterol dropped to 170, my thyroid tested normal. The most exciting change was **my B-12 tested normal for the first time in many years and my doctor said I don't need B-12 shots any more**. I love how I feel! The murmurs stopped. I have a lot less cravings for unhealthy foods. I lost 12 pounds and it feels so good, especially because I am a dancer. I eat two meals a day and have a lot of energy. I dance swing and polka ten hours a week vigorously. My white hair of twenty years is suddenly growing dark again.

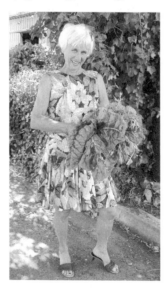

At 67 years old I don't fear anything anymore as my life attitude has significantly changed. I've never felt so well balanced in my whole life! My massage therapist told me my skin is glowing and my muscle tone has improved. I look ten years younger and I feel twenty years younger. Since I incorporated green smoothies into my diet my kids can't keep up with me any more and I beat my seventeen-year-old grandson in tennis. At our dance club I out-dance a lot of younger dancers. I can do six hours straight of Polka, Waltzes or Swing. People always ask me what is my secret. Since I carry my green drink everywhere I am always happy to share.

Many people of my age often have severe digestion problems, which I suffered also. Since I began drinking green smoothies my bowels work fantastically; one meal in, one meal out. My kidneys became a lot stronger, I don't wake up to urinate in the middle of the night anymore. My liver spots have faded noticeably. My eyesight improved so that I don't need my glasses most of the time. I am able to maintain a positive attitude even through the most challenging moments of my life. I feel calmer and more focused. I recently increased my business in Washington D.C which I run from California, three thousand miles away, using fax, computer, phone, and frequently commute by plane. I also host seven huge potlucks per year with the San Francisco Vegetarian Society and East Bay Vegetarian Society as well as many raw food potlucks and classes. To help other people with healing information I maintain my own website. www.LizzysLanding.com

I am supporting Victoria's research on chimpanzees and everything else she is involved in. I believe that the raw diet with green smoothies added is the future of all nutrition. I admire Victoria's courage and purpose of life to make a healthier planet.   — *Elizabeth Bechtold, CA*

Healing Eczema

I am 57 years old and I have been very allergic since childhood to everything. I was born with eczema and had to take heavy medications all my life. Every night I would scratch my entire body till it was raw and bleeding. I got worse and worse and the doctors doubled my medication including steroids. It put out some of the fire but left bleeding and bruised with ugly rashes all over. I was hospitalized five times for several days which never helped. Three times I felt so ill that I thought I would die.

The miracle began when my friend Elizabeth introduced me to a so called "green smoothie." This remarkable beverage not only greatly improved my skin condition, but I am also sleeping much better — with out scratching myself bloody every night. After only two weeks I truly am feeling more comfortable in my skin, looking better every day. This is a blessing which I cannot fully express in words. **My endless hell is now coming to an end.** It is truly a blessing to feel better and to finally become more productive in my life after 57 years of suffering. Thank you Elizabeth and Victoria.

— *Karl E. U. from California*

❧

Reversing Pancreatic Cancer

I am a middle school teacher of English in Taipei, Taiwan, with a very stressful life. As a result of my annual physical exam, I was told that I had pancreatic cancer, as the CE190 test came at a level of 40. Normal is 33. I felt scared and didn't want to die. I have two daughters who are still in school and entirely depend on me. Instead of taking a traditional medical way, I tried drinking wheatgrass juice, but I couldn't tolerate the taste at all. I began to eat raw fruits and vegetables and stopped eating meat and dairy products. After three months, I was again tested. The test again came out with a level of 40. Doctors told me that my cancer was not progressing, but it was also not diminishing. Then I read Victoria's book and learned about green smoothies. I began drinking 16 ounces of the green smoothies daily, and they became a regular part of my daily diet. I usually used orange juice as liquid, added a banana, and pineapple or mango. The green was parsley, sunflower sprouts, romaine lettuce and young pea sprouts. After another three months, when I returned to do my follow up check-up, the CE190 test showed a level of 28, better than normal! I believe that the **green smoothies saved my life**. — *S. Chiao, Taiwan*

Green Smoothies Help a Family Become Raw Fooders

I am a certified herbalist and have helped a lot of people with their health through consultations in my home and classes I have taught. After the birth of my 6th child, my health started to decline. Even though I had knowledge of herbs I was not able to help myself feel well. With my own health poor, I gave up doing the classes and cut back on my clients. Most of my life I have been a very energetic person, so when my energy started to decline I turned to caffeine to give myself a temporary lift. My blood sugar was so off that I had to eat constantly. Eating became a chore that I no longer enjoyed. I suffered from insomnia, dandruff, exhaustion, worry, depression, junk food cravings, and bad moods.

When I first heard about Victoria's class, I was reluctant to go. I did end up going and took a few friends with me. We all liked the smoothies a lot. Everything Victoria taught about greens fit with what I already knew. I started making the smoothies the next morning, out of wild greens from my yard. My family liked the smoothies too, so I started to make a gallon a day for them. Then I was able to get in on the study that Victoria and Dr. Fieber did. I started to tell all my friends about the smoothies.

Raw Family was sitting on my hutch and I was avoiding reading it. My husband picked it up and read it. Then he told me that I should read it. I did and realized that this was story was remarkable. I felt hope that my health would be restored.

After reading *Raw Family* my husband was interested in going raw but had understandable concerns. The main one was that he had never seen a vegetarian man who looked strong and healthy. My husband likes to work out and he did not want to go raw if he was going to lose muscle mass. When Igor dropped off smoothies, my husband was able to meet him. Igor likes to workout. Actually he owns about 300 different workout machines. He was also trained in massage in Moscow. My husband was impressed with how healthy Igor's skin looked and how well built he was.

My opinion is that **being a raw vegetarian is a big difference from being a cooked food vegetarian**. I do not think a person gets enough protein from eating cooked vegetables. The raw foodists are the only people I have seen who have a truly healthy look to them.

The first thing that the smoothies did for me was help me not crave junk food. I think bad cravings are from nutritional deficiencies. When those deficiencies are met, then the cravings go away. We should always listen to our cravings. That is one of the first questions I ask clients when they come to see me. I think smoothies are a key factor in more people becoming raw. If a person is not dealing with constant cravings, then they will find being raw a lot easier.

When I stopped craving junk food, I realized I really did want to go raw. As I progressed toward being raw my family and friends watched me. One friend even told me that, "We are going to let you be the guinea pig for all this and we will watch how it turns out for you before we become raw." Well, it has turned out great and most of them are going raw now too. This includes my husband and 6 children, the oldest being 15.

I have my energy back! I sleep soundly through the night. About 5 a.m. I wake up on my own, feeling rested and ready for the day. My emotions are balancing out; I am positive, no longer crave caffeine, and have an overall feeling of well-being. I finally lost the last 10 pounds that I had gained from pregnancy. Actually some days I feel so good I can only describe it as feeling like I am high on drugs. I think that we were created by God to feel that good all the time. That is why people like drugs so much because somewhere inside us we desire to feel the way God created us to be.

I have had some detox days, but I just take it easy on those days and allow myself to heal. I just keep telling myself that I am getting rid of trash that might have caused more illness in the long run. My husband is also a support at those times and tells me, "You know this diet is right; just hang in there."

My husband has always needed a lot of sleep but he is able to get by with 5 hours at times now. My children are all getting along better. My 15 year old says she is smarter. My 12 year old has more energy and her dandruff and acne is clearing up.

Thank you, Victoria for changing my life, and the life of my family and friends with your enthusiastic sharing about raw foods. I pray the Lord richly blesses you for it.

— Angela R.

Indigestion and Cravings for Sweets are Gone

Dear Sister Victoria,

Audrey's and my (Hugh) experiences are very similar with the "Green Smoothies":

1. We have each, dropped about 5 pounds since starting this regimen a couple of months ago. Audrey went from 150 down to 145, and Hugh from 196 down to 191, approximately.

2. We are experiencing great energy, along with free and wonderful bowel movements — often three times daily! ☺

3. According to the "acid tests," Audrey (blood type "O–") has plenty of stomach acid, naturally, and hardly ever experiences indigestion. Hugh (blood type "A+") has very low stomach acid, (I took the four acid capsules, even, with my "regular full meal," and they did the trick with no indigestion, from lack of acid, and no "burning" from too much acid! I used to have indigestion every day depending upon

baking soda for comfort for a long time, then I discovered if I ate a whole orange at the first onset of indigestion, it would be gone by the time I finished eating said orange! That being as it may — with the "green smoothies" I experience no stomach discomforts of any kind! It's wonderful!

4. Our **desire for ice-cream and sweets has dwindled FAST!** A nice, juicy steak sounds good — and I may salivate a bit thinking of it — but I have no problem in passing it up, either. I, Hugh, confess that twice in the past two weeks, we were invited to steak bar-b-ques, and twice I went off the wagon — AND, twice I suffered with indigestion afterward! It's just not worth it! After last evening's feast of RAW FOOD at our first Raw Food Potluck in Myrtle Creek, I ate like a pig, after, first, having a Green Smoothie before we left home for said Potluck, and still did not experience any indigestion, whatsoever.

We are BELIEVERS! AND, we are definite disciples of one Victoria Boutenko, and our own "Dr. Paul." You both are beautiful people and we are so fortunate to know and experience you and your teachings.   — *Hugh and Audrey B.*

Green Smoothies Provide Relief from Cravings for Too Much Fats

We are two women in our forties. One of us was 100 percent raw for 2 years and is now about 75 percent raw vegetarian; the other is about 40 percent raw and eats meat. We began drinking green smoothies about 2 months ago after reading Victoria's article *Ode to Green Smoothies*. We noticed a couple of things right away: they taste GREAT! We found that not only were we surprised by their delicious flavor, but also we began to crave them. We felt happy having two of our meals per day consist of green smoothies. The "40 percent raw" one of us began losing weight effortlessly and wanted only green smoothies for two meals (and sometimes every meal). The "75 percent raw" one of us had a healing crisis after a 5-day cleanse with just green smoothies and fruit. We feel the green smoothies are a wonderful way to get relief from cravings for too much raw fats: **the smoothies are so satisfying and fat free**. We feel we are on the road to even better health! Thank you!

— *MA & LC in Berkeley, CA*

Given up Coffee

I went through a divorce last year and have been under quite a bit of stress. When I attended the first raw food lecture, I had been really stressed out. My digestion had gotten so bad that almost everything I ate caused gas, bloating. My doctor said I was deficient in almost everything because I wasn't absorbing much of anything. So, when I was able to participate in the study I was thrilled. When we first started the study, I didn't notice any difference when I got up to the 4 capsules of HCL with food. I know I have very little stomach acid and have a hard time digesting. When we started on the smoothies, I often had to use 1 capsule of HCL just to keep from having what I guessed is heart burn or acid reflux if I was at all stressed. With that, I could digest the smoothie just fine. I didn't notice much the first week but starting the second week I was amazed. I started waking up before my alarm went off, and that was really something.

Usually I could barely wake up and drag myself out of bed even after 8 hours of sleep. I was waking up easily and ready to start my day after that. I hadn't given up all my bad habits like coffee in the morning, cooked and raw foods, and some wine at night. Even with doing those "bad" things my energy was much better.

I really started looking forward to the smoothies every day and would have loved to have had more. I just didn't have the time right then to make more of it for myself. Being a single mom, I work too many hours trying to build my business, and still have to work at a part-time job. I'm trying to spend quality time with my son too, so find that having enough time at home is a challenge for me. Now that school is out and my son's activities have slowed down a bit, I am able to be at home more so plan to get myself back into the routine of having green smoothies every day. I know I felt so much better and had more energy. **I have given up coffee now and have turned my coffee grinder into my flax seed grinder**. I also noticed that my colon was working better while I was doing the smoothies. So, that really helped me feel less toxic as well. Eating raw is something I KNOW is the right thing to do; I just have a hard time making it happen. I think that **doing the smoothies makes it easier than ever to do the raw thing** and to get the nutrients that I am lacking in. My digestion is gradually improving and I did lose 2# during the month study. Not a huge weight loss, but a loss nonetheless. I wonder how much I would have lost if I hadn't been doing all the "bad" things at the same time! I needed this push to get back into taking better care of myself, so I thank you for that. Busy moms need better self-care, doing the green smoothies is how I'm going to do that! I'm looking forward to seeing my health continue to improve and my energy increase. I want to keep up with this teenage boy of mine! :o)

Thank you, Thank you! I look forward to seeing you and your family again. God Bless You!   — L.H.

Cataract Regressed from 40% to 10%

Dear Victoria,

We met in May at Super Sprouts in Toronto. Thank you for a most information loaded session and the support that you provide to so many health seekers, including my family and myself.

On October of 2004 I was told that my cholesterol level was so high, it was even a miracle that I was able to go to the doctor's office to hear this terrible news.

Parallel to that, arthritis in both my hands was so painful that every morning I was waking up with aches and pains from my crippling hands. I was devastated since I play the piano, and music is a great part of my life.

To top it all, my eyesight was getting worse, and a cataract was setting into my left eye. The eye doctor told me that this was a progressive illness and only surgery would help. . . .

What to do then? more pills . . . NO . . . I decided with the help of RAW friends to go RAW immediately. . . . I was going on a trip to Germany and had no doubts that I would survive following the RAW diet. My family overseas had prepared all kinds of cooked foods and baked cakes for my arrival. I announced to them that, on doctor's orders, I had to continue RAW... a big silence followed... but to my amazement, they all respected my wish. I even prepared delicious RAW foods, including desserts. Everyone was astounded and more than pleasantly surprised at the newly discovered taste.

I spent 4 weeks overseas, using the recipes that I had taken with me to keep me going. I had a ball everywhere.

I got back and went back for another check up. The doctor announced to me that my cholesterol was incredibly good, compared to that of a young person (I am 58 years young... and that was another compliment) — he said, whatever I was doing was good, to keep on doing it. I share with him my experience with the RAW diet, but that went in one ear and out the other....

Then I went for my eye examination and the eye doctor was totally taken aback when he announced to me that **not only had the cataract regressed from 40% to 10%, but my eyesight was getting much better and I needed new prescription glasses** now. I asked him then if he has in all his years of practice had a similar case, and his answer was an emphatic NO. I then told him that I credited this improvement and reversal of sickness to my RAW diet. It didn't click with him, but the patients in the waiting room all heard what I shared with my doctor. It was amazing that he did not connect at all ... may be later... but this is bad for his business, right?

Anyway, I have thrown out all my pills since last October, and I feel so much better now. My energy level is so much higher; I have lost 35 lbs and never looked so good in my life before.

These are the tangible results after a few months of RAW diet, I'm wondering the wonderful rejuvenation my internal organs also must experience . . . .

Thank you, Victoria for your courage to have wanted to prove the medical community wrong, and to show the healthier alternative to cooked foods and pills (Yeah!)

Keep smiling and healthy,

— *Deanna A. Gontard, May 25th, 2005*

Happy Days on Raw Foods

Before Victoria and Igor's presentation in Riddle, I was in a very sad place. I didn't want to be on the planet anymore. I felt so tired, so depressed, so sick. When I heard the enthusiastic presentation by Victoria my heart smiled. I found new hope. I found an answer to my problems! I felt inside that eating more fresh fruits and vegetables and greens was right for me, exactly what I needed. But I didn't know how — or if I could do it.

I had so little stomach acid that I was part of the green study. Thank you! 30 days on green smoothies and my body wants only raw foods. I feel energy! My vision began to improve and my joy came back!

My blood sugars stabilized. My moods stabilized. I want to live! I have energy! I have regular bowel movements. My vision is clearer. My skin is healthier. I feel so grateful! Thank you.   — *Bridget BW, June 14, 2005*

Raw Food Baby Zander

Arrival of Z:

Alexander (alias Zander, alias Z) Graff Levin, born in Beaufort, SC, January 1, 2004, six pounds and thirteen ounces, 19.50 inches long. We received the call to come get [adopt] Zander when he was four days old; the lawyer had been out of town on vacation when Z was born.

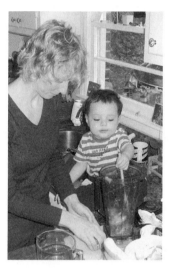

First–Forth months. Z's main foods: goat milk, breast milk from a wet nurse, water.

Fifth month. We introduced Z to raw food juices.

Sixth month. Added barley green juice, as well as thinly blended green smoothies in small amounts.

Ninth month. Z loves avocados and apples

Tenth month. Z prefers to have lemons, apples and celery in every smoothie.

Eleventh month. **Blood iron count: 12.9!** Z likes to help me in the kitchen when I make smoothies. He sits on the countertop and hands me things [not by name yet], or I let him stir the contents of the blender [unplugged] with a large wooden spoon. It was suggested that I increase Z's iron supply. So, with more greens added [lettuce and parsley] and a bit of Vital K and Floradix herbal combinations, Z's blood was tested at a high 12.9%! Z's doctor said, "Wow! What have you been feeding him, nails?"

Twelfth month. Z began to eat 'green-based' smoothies. Z likes to try feeding himself, and then offers it to us on his spoon. Z still wants milk, and nearly weaned himself. But, started again when I was gone for a few days.

Fifteenth and sixteenth months. Z's blood count remains high. Per my request, it was last tested April 2005 at a level of 11.9. Z's pediatrician asked a lot of questions during the last visit. Every answer was resoundingly positive to his ears. The doctor's final words were, "**Everything checks out at or above normal.** I don't need to recheck him until the 24 month, well-patient visit." This means that he recommended skipping the routine 18 month old check up.

Z is walking everywhere, and we are raising things to new levels in the house to keep out of Z's lengthening arms. He says random phrases by now, such as: "I'm okay," "What you doin'?," "How're you doin'?" I don't know," "I love you," "bye-bye," "thank you," "I do it" and "I didn't do it."

A few more things:

1. Since his introduction to green food, until now, Z has had two or three regular bowel movements each day. I'm convinced that the green-based smoothies are keeping his bowels lubricated and hydrated, mostly because of the high water and oil contents. The fruit and veggie fiber also stimulates peristalsis.

4. I like the old adage, "Let food be your medicine and medicine be your food."

Go ahead and use my name. Thanks for asking.

— *Clare Levin, clare@classictouch.net*

Little Nicolas Likes It Too!

I started drinking "green smoothies" along with my husband Stephan religiously when I was about 6 months pregnant with our son Nicolas, the first grandson of the

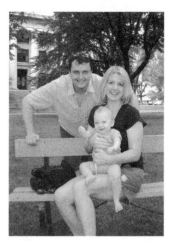

Boutenko family. I noticed that I had more energy and had an overall feeling of good health. I also had a wonderful delivery that went smoothly and the baby did not exhibit the usual signs of distress during contractions such as a low heart beat. In fact, every time a contraction started, the baby's heartbeat would not faulter in the slightest. After Nicolas was born, I continued the smoothies of which I believe the benefits through breast-feeding went directly to him. He has amazed all of us including his pediatrician because he is consistently ahead of the curve in the developmental stages and is now trying to walk. Now Nicolas is almost 9 months old and unlike his peers, has never been sick once. We credit our excellent health to the green smoothie.

— *Tasia, Stephan and Nicolas Boutenko*

Testimonials of Roseburg Study Participants

To collect more data for my research, I asked the participants of the Roseburg study to answer the following questions.

1. Was it hard to drink one quart of Green Smoothie every day?
2. Did the rest of your diet change as a result of the green smoothies?
3. Did you notice any changes in your health?
4. Did your cravings for unhealthy foods lessen?
5. Have you noticed any change in your weight?
6. Did your sleep change?
7. Did your elimination change?
8. Did your energy change?
9. Did anybody comment on how you looked?
10. Did you have any symptoms of detox?
11. Did you have any negative experiences?
12. Would you like to continue drinking Green Smoothies?

The answers were so authentic that I decided to include them all in order to reflect the multitude of positive changes that occurred. I took out only the un-answered questions.

❦ Hugh B.

1. Was it hard to drink one quart of Green Smoothie every day?
No.

2. Did the rest of your diet change as a result of the green smoothies?
Yes. I have less desire for other foods!

3. Did you notice any changes in your health?
Yes. More energy.

4. Did your cravings for unhealthy foods lessen?
Yes. Less ice cream these days.

5. Have you noticed any change in your weight?
Yes. Slight loss (4 lbs).

6. Did your sleep change?
Yes. Much.

7. Did your elimination change?
Oh yes!

8. Did anybody comment on how you looked?
No. Not to my face, anyway! ☹

9. Did you have any symptoms of detox?
Not that I can tell — maybe that's why I'm so tired today.

10. Did you have any negative experiences?
No negatives.

11. Would you like to continue drinking Green Smoothies?
Yes. Plan to do so! Great sex.

❦ A. R.

1. Was it hard to drink one quart of Green Smoothie every day?
No, I drank more and loved them. Family started drinking also and get upset if I do not make smoothies for them.

2. Did the rest of your diet change as a result of the green smoothies?
Yes, it made me want to eat raw and so I am now 95% raw. I have not craved junk.

3. Did you notice any changes in your health?

Yes, I am sleeping well, I have energy, I am positive, I lost 10 lbs, dandruff healed.

4. Did your cravings for unhealthy foods lessen?

Yes, I am not craving junk!

5. Have you noticed any change in your weight?

Yes, lost 10 pounds but was also raw.

6. Did your sleep change?

Sleep great! I have had problems with insomnia for years.

7. Did your energy change?

I have great energy. I get up at 5 a.m. and feel rested and energetic.

Increased sex drive.

8. Did anybody comment on how you looked?

Yes. Husband and children. I can see a glow on my own face.

9. Did you have any negative experiences?

Only the mild detox but I was willing to do it because of the reward.

10. Would you like to continue drinking Green Smoothies?

Yes, my whole family is hooked.

Thank you so much. I think that the green smoothies are one of the most nutritious things we can ingest. I have been telling my family and friends about it. You have played a part in totally changing my life!

❀ T. T.

1. Was it hard to drink one quart of Green Smoothie every day?

No! Very enjoyable, wanted more.

2. Did the rest of your diet change as a result of the green smoothies?

Wasn't as hungry — wanted less coffee.

3. Did you notice any changes in your health?

Had more energy.

4. Did your sleep change?

Yes, I slept better, longer without waking

5. Did your energy change?

I used to have lows around 2 pm every day. Now I only have those around once a week or so.

6. Did you have any symptoms of detox?

Noticed no side effects.

7. Would you like to continue drinking Green Smoothies?

Will make my own smoothies and ENJOY my way to better health. Am thinking about selling Green Smoothies at my shop.

❧ T. W.

1. Was it hard to drink one quart of Green Smoothie every day?

No! Actually I got used to drinking smoothies and after a week, actually wanted a smoothie.

2. Did the rest of your diet change as a result of the green smoothies?

Yes. I ate less food at each meal.

3. Did you notice any changes in your health?

Yes. I had more energy and did not take as many afternoon naps. I also did not get hunger pangs before meals and did not get a sugar low in the afternoon.

4. Did your cravings for unhealthy foods lessen?

A little bit.

5. Have you noticed any change in your weight?

Weight stayed about the same — have been working on our yard (5 acres) so already had weight loss.

6. Did your sleep change?

Yes, right from the first days I slept very soundly and did not grind my teeth at night.

7. Did your elimination change?

My elimination doubled! Usually I was only once a day — now twice a day very regularly.

8. Did your energy change?

Definite increase in energy — was able to work in the yard and garden all day with just a couple of breaks. Before I had to take an afternoon nap all the time.

9. Did anybody comment on how you looked?

We really did not see anyone else, however we did feel much better.

10. Did you have any symptoms of detox?

Yes, stomach cramps on the second round of green smoothies. Very bloated with the first couple of days — after that, no problem.

11. Did you have any negative experiences?

No other negative effects.

12. Would you like to continue drinking Green Smoothies?

Yes, will continue drinking green smoothies — enjoy the flavor and better health — they are a part of my daily routine.

❀ L. C.

1. Was it hard to drink one quart of Green Smoothie every day?

No. Eat it for breakfast, harder at night. Can't eat a lot and drink also.

2. Did the rest of your diet change as a result of the green smoothies?

Eating more raw. Trying to find food that is like things I like or crave, bread, cheese.

3. Did your cravings for unhealthy foods lessen?

No, some things I wanted badly, textures, flavors, warmth, heat, familiar. Used to drink coffee, now do not.

4. Have you noticed any change in your weight?

Lost 4–5 lbs.

5. Did your sleep change?

I sleep sounder. Don't get up as often.

6. Did your elimination change?

Definitely regular. Am going more frequently.

7. Did your energy change?

Better energy. I used to get tired at 2–3 in the afternoon. Took supplements, drank coffee, I don't get tired now unless I'm eating more cooked food.

8. Did anybody comment on how you looked?

Yes, looked glowing.

9. Did you have any symptoms of detox?

Headaches. Fever, flu, bad cold, bronchitis in the beginning.

10. Did you have any negative experiences?

Learning to cook raw, using equipment not familiar with. Need food that's fast and easy.

11. Would you like to continue drinking Green Smoothies?

Yes. I'm calmer, more peaceful, less anxious.

❧ L. M.

1. Was it hard to drink one quart of Green Smoothie every day?

No (More! I made some of my own.)

2. Did the rest of your diet change as a result of the green smoothies?

Yes. Made more smoothies and ate less dessert and others, less carbs.

3. Did you notice any changes in your health?

Yes. More energy and lost weight.

4. Did your cravings for unhealthy foods lessen?

Yes.

5. Have you noticed any change in your weight?

Yes. Lost 9–11 lbs.

6. Did your sleep change?

Sleep better a little.

7. Did your elimination change?

I urinate more. Less constipated

8. Did your energy change?

More energy.

9. Did anybody comment on how you looked?

Yes.

10. Did you have any symptoms of detox?

Maybe mild flu in the beginning.

11. Did you have any negative experiences?

No.

12. Would you like to continue drinking Green Smoothies?

Yes!

❀ Rebeca S.

1. Was it hard to drink one quart of Green Smoothie every day?

No, I wish I could have more a day.

2. Did the rest of your diet change as a result of the green smoothies?

Yes, I stopped craving sugars and carbohydrates.

3. Did you notice any changes in your health?

Yes, I feel more energy and no more constipation it is great!

4. Did your cravings for unhealthy foods lessen?

Yes.

5. Have you noticed any change in your weight?

No, definitively no, I am not 100% raw food yet.

6. Did your sleep change?

My sleeping is much better.

7. Did your elimination change?

My bowel movement is great now!.

8. Did your energy change?

Yes, I have a lot more energy.

9. Did anybody comment on how you looked?

No, nobody.

10. Did you have any symptoms of detox?

Only itching. Irregular itching all over my body during first week.

11. Did you have any negative experiences?

No.

12. Would you like to continue drinking Green Smoothies?

Yes, absolutely positive.

Thank you, very much I appreciate everything all of your family has been doing for us.

❧ Brent G.

1. Was it hard to drink one quart of Green Smoothie every day?

At first.

2. Did the rest of your diet change as a result of the green smoothies?

Somewhat, less milk and meat.

3. Did you notice any changes in your health?

Less fatigue, more energy.

4. Did your cravings for unhealthy foods lessen?

Yes, except coffee.

5. Have you noticed any change in your weight?

No.

6. Did your sleep change?

Yes. Get up earlier, less trips to the bathroom.

7. Did your elimination change?

Bowel movement improved.

8. Did your energy change?

Ability to work longer.

9. Did anybody comment on how you looked?

Yes, said I looked less stressed.

10. Did you have any symptoms of detox?

Some, headache, more acne.

11. Did you have any negative experiences?
No.

12. Would you like to continue drinking Green Smoothies?
Yes.

Carrie M.

1. Was it hard to drink one quart of Green Smoothie every day?
No. Easy.

2. Did the rest of your diet change as a result of the green smoothies?
Yes. Eating all raw.

3. Did you notice any changes in your health?
Yes. Less feeling disoriented when it has been several hours since eating.

4. Did your cravings for unhealthy foods lessen?
Yes. No cravings.

5. Have you noticed any change in your weight?
Yes. Lost 5 lbs. in first two weeks. No loss this past week.

6. Did your sleep change?
Maybe a little better, but basically the same.

7. Did your elimination change?
Yes. More frequently, about five times a day.

8. Did your energy change?
A little more energy, mind a little clearer.

9. Did you have any symptoms of detox?
Only all the trips to the bathroom. Felt bad one afternoon.

10. Did you have any negative experiences?
No.

11. Would you like to continue drinking Green Smoothies?
Will continue due to a positive blood test on the ANA test.

🌺 **Mandy O.** (mom answering for her)

1. Was it hard to drink one quart of Green Smoothie every day?
No.

2. Did you notice any changes in your health?
Yes. Less asthma — breathing a lot easier than her twin sister who didn't take smoothie (see below).

3. Have you noticed any change in your weight?
Was 113 lbs, now 110 because it filled her up.

4. Did your energy change?
Yes. Ability to run longer without being out of breath.

5. Did you have any symptoms of detox?
No.

Mandy and Becky are identical twins. 17 years old. Both are very active and soccer stars. Mandy drank the green smoothie. Becky did not. Before starting, Mandy had severe asthma attacks — first in four years. (They were 5 weeks premature) Mandy has had lung problems since birth — Becky does not.)

One week after starting green smoothie Mandy's asthma attacks stopped. After week 2 they started running to get a jump start for fall soccer. The first time they ran — 1 mile — Becky huffed and puffed like their friends running with them during and after the run. Mandy had very little trouble breathing during and after the run. She felt she was breathing easier and deeper even up the hill. They run twice a week after school. Becky huffs and puff after, Mandy does not. Becky caught what was going around school — illness. Mandy did not.

🌺 **LaVee H.**

1. Was it hard to drink one quart of Green Smoothie every day?
No. I would have liked to be using more. It was so nice to have the work done for me. Thank you!

2. Did the rest of your diet change as a result of the green smoothies?

Yes. I was more conscious of eating more raw food each day.

3. Did you notice any changes in your health?

Yes. I had more energy, am waking up before alarm goes off.

4. Did your cravings for unhealthy foods lessen?

Sometimes — stress influenced this craving more than anything.

5. Have you noticed any change in your weight?

Yes. I lost almost 2 lbs.

6. Did your sleep change?

Yes. I dream more, wake before alarm goes off. (I usually sleep ok.)

7. Did your elimination change?

Yes, Less constipated — started more green, then went to more brown.

8. Did your energy change?

Yes. More energy — woke up easier in the morning — happier

9. Did anybody comment on how you looked?

Yes. One person said I looked good.

10. Did you have any symptoms of detox?

Yes. Slight nausea or heartburn — usually happened when I was extremely stressed before drinking the smoothie. I have been going through a lot of emotional things that have been very stressful, so maybe I was detoxing negative emotions more than physical detox.

11. Would you like to continue drinking Green Smoothies?

Yes. I hope to do even more.

❧ Audrey B.

1. Was it hard to drink one quart of Green Smoothie every day?

No, Easy, delicious.

2. Did the rest of your diet change as a result of the green smoothies?

Yes. Cut back a lot and watched what we ate.

3. Did you notice any changes in your health?

Yes. The green smoothie cleared my system daily.

4. Did your cravings for unhealthy foods lessen?

Yes. We are working on eliminating ice cream.

5. Have you noticed any change in your weight?

Yes. Loss — 4 lbs.

6. Did your sleep change?

Yes. Slept better and a deeper sleep.

7. Did your elimination change?

Yes. You get up — walk and have to go.

8. Did your energy change?

Yes. I'm pleased.

9. Did anybody comment on how you looked?

Yes. I was told I was glowing. Sex life improved.

10. Did you have any symptoms of detox?

No symptoms that I felt.

11. Did you have any negative experiences?

No. None at all.

12. Would you like to continue drinking Green Smoothies?

Yes. Definitely plan to do so!

❧ Marion C., age 75

1. Was it hard to drink one quart of Green Smoothie every day?

No problem drinking 1 qt. daily. Sometimes mixed other fruit juice with.

2. Did the rest of your diet change as a result of the green smoothies?

With smoothies I take one glass in a.m. early, one about noon, and again eve. or bedtime.

3. Did you notice any changes in your health?

Have noticed no craving for any food. Also notice fingernails are stronger again.

4. Did your cravings for unhealthy foods lessen?

Yes. Usually I have had one meal and smoothies kept me satisfied.

5. Have you noticed any change in your weight?

No weight change. Never has been.

6. Did your sleep change?

Sleep more soundly now. Before, may lay for 2–3 hours before getting to sleep. Used Valerian Root capsules too.

7. Did your elimination change?

Bowels have always been very loose and pale yellow color. Now they are soft and may go 3 X daily. No abdominal discomfort.

8. Did your energy change?

Used to need rest in p.m. Now can keep busy all day with occasional breaks so seems like more energy. Activities — Caring for goats/llamas. Gardening, spreading crushed rock and wood chips for landscaping. Definitely more energy.

9. Did you have any symptoms of detox?

No. No bad reaction whatever.

10. Did you have any negative experiences?

No.

11. Would you like to continue drinking Green Smoothies?

I have had some heart arrhythmia for several years, and taking multifood supplements. Am taking Mannatech food supplements since Dec. 2004 and have noticed heart rhythm back to normal. Also have had cold hands and feet, minimal energy, but all these minor problems have disappeared.

Have always thought that I may be hypothyroid but something I'm doing is good, so, I am happy, and plan to remain on smoothies.

❧ Gabrielle R., age 35

1. Was it hard to drink one quart of Green Smoothie every day?

    Yes, I did have to break into small portions, taste was fine, but I did have trouble with thickness and quantity as well as too little variety, but I will experiment on my own.

2. Did the rest of your diet change as a result of the green smoothies?

    Yes, I ate less in general. I craved less "junk food" and more fruits and raw foods.

3. Did you notice any changes in your health?

    Yes, more energy! I require less sleep, my temperament is more even and pleasant; I had none of my usual "PMS" symptoms and my skin cleared up beautifully.

4. Did your cravings for unhealthy foods lessen?

    Yes. I was able to drop many unhealthy items from my diet fairly easily.

5. Have you noticed any change in your weight?

    I only lost less than 5 lbs by the scale, but I do feel as thought I lost a bit more.

6. Did your sleep change?

    I sleep better, and require less per night. I wake up fully awake and don't linger in bed as I used to.

7. Did your elimination change?

    I definitely go more than ever before and I definitely am urinating more frequently. I didn't notice any specific color changes.

8. Did your energy change?

Yes. I find each evening, that everything I set out to do each day actually got done! I don't have work piled up undone at the end of the day as I would before.

9. Did anybody comment on how you looked?

I did have just a couple of mild compliments.

10. Did you have any symptoms of detox?

I did have mild mucus coughing and through sinuses, also mild nausea the first few days.

11. Did you have any negative experiences?

No!

12. Would you like to continue drinking Green Smoothies?

Definitely. I look forward to experimenting with various recipes and sharing them with my family.

🌿 Leah W.

1. Was it hard to drink one quart of Green Smoothie every day?

No, however I wouldn't want more.

2. Did the rest of your diet change as a result of the green smoothies?

I did eat more veggies as I was more aware of "good" foods.

3. Did you notice any changes in your health?

No constipation at all, fresher taste in foods, possibly more energy.

4. Did your cravings for unhealthy foods lessen?

It filled me up so that I ate less other foods, but could still desire other foods.

5. Did your elimination change?

Usually have 1 BM per day but with smoothies I had 2 or more with no constipation.

6. Did your energy change?

Before smoothie I would eat dinner then sit and watch

T.V. and fall asleep. After smoothie I didn't fall asleep watching T.V.

7. Would you like to continue drinking Green Smoothies?
Yes! I will try to continue and experiment with different greens, adding more organic produce as well.

Thank you so much for exposing me to raw foods, greens and better nutrition! You're great!.

Al C.

1. Was it hard to drink one quart of Green Smoothie every day?
No, I could do more easily.

2. Did the rest of your diet change as a result of the green smoothies?
Yes. I've started to eat a lot more salads but I occasionally still get cravings.

3. Did you notice any changes in your health?
I've lost about 5–6 pounds.

4. Did your cravings for unhealthy foods lessen?
I seem to eat far less junk.

5. Have you noticed any change in your weight?
I've lost about 5–6 pounds.

6. Did your sleep change?
I seem to toss and turn less as my hair isn't as messy in the morning when I wake up.

7. Did your elimination change?
3 to 4 times daily. Felt like whole colon was emptying all at once.

8. Did your energy change?
Not a really noticeable change yet — seems about the same.

9. Did you have any negative experiences?
No.

10. Would you like to continue drinking Green Smoothies?

I will continue, yes.

I am 54. I definitely noticed a significant improvement in my male response — about 15 years worth.

❦ Wib

1. Did the rest of your diet change as a result of the green smoothies?

Yes, less prepared food.

2. Did you notice any changes in your health?

Yes. 3 lbs. weight loss

3. Did your cravings for unhealthy foods lessen?

Yes. Maybe motivational rather than taste.

4. Did your sleep change?

Yes, rested more consistently.

5. Did your elimination change?

Bowel more regular, urine more sensational

6. Did you have any symptoms of detox?

Mild headaches.

7. Did you have any negative experiences?

Never did enjoy the taste, just drank for test and health's sake.

8. Would you like to continue drinking Green Smoothies?

Yes. In various degrees and kinds of drinks and preparations. We will not be going 100% raw, hopefully 75–90% raw. But thanks for your focus and help.

❦ Dee S.

1. Was it hard to drink one quart of Green Smoothie every day?

No.

2. Did the rest of your diet change as a result of the green smoothies?

Yes, ate mostly raw.

3. Did your cravings for unhealthy foods lessen?

Yes.

4. Have you noticed any change in your weight?

Yes, lost 10 lbs.

5. Did anybody comment on how you looked?

A few people noticed weight loss.

6. Did you have any symptoms of detox?

Not that I was aware of.

7. Did you have any negative experiences?

Nothing negative.

❧ Terri B., age 51

1. Was it hard to drink one quart of Green Smoothie every day?

No. It was easy and enjoyable. More would have been nice.

2. Did the rest of your diet change as a result of the green smoothies?

Yes, my family and myself have started eating some raw.

3. Did you notice any changes in your health?

Yes, I have more energy and my husband is easier to get along with.

4. Did your cravings for unhealthy foods lessen?

Yes, my cravings are almost gone. When having a lot of bad choices available, I didn't care and did not eat.

5. Have you noticed any change in your weight?

Yes, I have lost 18–20 lbs.

6. Did your sleep change?

I was rested, but I did get up more often to use the restroom to urinate.

7. Did your elimination change?

Yes, I eliminated a lot more than I consumed, and it was easy and gentle.

8. Did your energy change?

Yes, I no longer desire a nap whenever time is available.

9. Did you have any symptoms of detox?

Yes. Burning of eyes, and lips, headaches.

10. Did you have any negative experiences?

No — It has been a very positive. We are starting to go raw. And trying to figure out how to prepare for 6 people (4 of them being growing boys) is a bit overwhelming.

11. Would you like to continue drinking Green Smoothies?

Yes.

🌺 Berta D.

1. Was it hard to drink one quart of Green Smoothie every day?

No.

2. Did the rest of your diet change as a result of the green smoothies?

No. I think I crave sugar a little less.

3. Did you notice any changes in your health?

No. My weight is yo-yoing.

4. Did your energy change?

I'm walking a little more and I've joined Curves.

5. Did anybody comment on how you looked?

No one commented.

6. Did you have any symptoms of detox?

No.

7. Did you have any negative experiences?

No negative experiences.

8. Would you like to continue drinking Green Smoothies?

Have more positive than negative in all this experience.

🌿 Sunny D.

1. Was it hard to drink one quart of Green Smoothie every day?
No, not at all — I could drink them all day long.

2. Did you notice any changes in your health?
I noticed an improvement in my skin — especially on days when I did not eat other junk.

3. Did your cravings for unhealthy foods lessen?
A little bit — less interest in chocolate.

4. Have you noticed any change in your weight?
No, stayed the same.

5. Did your sleep change?
I sleep better, especially if I don't eat spicy food in addition to smoothies.

6. Did your elimination change?
A slight increase in volume.

7. Did your energy change?
Didn't notice a change in energy.

8. Did you have any symptoms of detox?
I had detox headaches for a night and a day.

9. Did you have any negative experiences?
None!

10. Would you like to continue drinking Green Smoothies?
Definitely! I had already been drinking a huge smoothie daily: 48 oz., approx. 75–80% fruit with some greens. I continued to drink that for this whole month in addition to the green smoothies. Now I will definitely be continuing the higher greens type smoothies — I would miss the greens too much if I stopped!

🌿 Cindy S.

1. Was it hard to drink one quart of Green Smoothie every day?
No — sometimes I wanted more

2. Did the rest of your diet change as a result of the green smoothies?

I wanted more fresh food — cooked food wasn't as appealing

3. Did you notice any changes in your health?

I was hungrier at meal times the first week or two. I had more regular bowel movements.

4. Did your cravings for unhealthy foods lessen?

Yes. I wasn't as hungry for sweets — I was more motivated to eat healthier.

5. Have you noticed any change in your weight?

I have lost some weight — I like it!

6. Did your sleep change?

I may be getting by with less sleep.

7. Did your elimination change?

I had more regular bowel movements — larger in size, and toward the end I noticed darker stools — perhaps getting rid of older accumulation?

8. Did your energy change?

I felt good knowing I was doing something so good for myself — my life is very busy and hectic — I'm sure if I were more disciplined, I would benefit more.

9. Did anybody comment on how you looked?

No one said anything except that my husband says I play the piano better now!

10. Did you have any symptoms of detox?

None that I know of.

11. Did you have any negative experiences?

None. I enjoyed very much being a part of this study and telling others about it.

12. Would you like to continue drinking Green Smoothies?

Yes. I want to keep this up.

✿ Vickie G. of Glide

1. Was it hard to drink one quart of Green Smoothie every day?

   At first, then got used to taste. Got easier, drinking more, want more.

2. Did the rest of your diet change as a result of the green smoothies?

   Some, occasionally more hungry.

3. Did you notice any changes in your health?

   Yes.

4. Did your cravings for unhealthy foods lessen?

   Yes. desire less chocolate and sweets at work.

5. Did your sleep change?

   Sleeping deeper, dreaming for the first time in almost a year.

6. Did your elimination change?

   More frequent. Used to have hard pebbles every time I went. Now larger, softer, still more frequent. Very thirsty now.

7. Did your energy change?

   Yes. Fewer naps/time. (I work 6 pm–6 am) More awake at work and alert, more energy at work.

8. Did anybody comment on how you looked?

   I did — less dark wrinkles under eyes and puffiness.

9. Did you have any symptoms of detox?

   Yes. Some headaches first weeks, now feel better. At first acid reflux went away, then had severe acid even in mouth, now no acid reflux.

10. Did you have any negative experiences?

    No.

11. Would you like to continue drinking Green Smoothies?

    Yes, desire to start own harvesting and doing own.
    At work, colds and flu go around and around, I usually got sick too. I haven't gotten sick since starting. Also my 5 year old drinks it too and likes it.

🌺 Bridget H.

1. Was it hard to drink one quart of Green Smoothie every day?
Very easy to drink, not hard at all to drink green smoothies.

2. Did the rest of your diet change as a result of the green smoothies?
My body wants raw foods starting around the 9th day of drinking green smoothies!
I want to be 100% raw foods soon!

3. Did you notice any changes in your health?
Increased energy, motivation to exercise more, my joy came back and my depression lifted and I don't have suicidal thoughts — less blood sugar fluctuations! Thank you!

4. Did your cravings for unhealthy foods lessen?
My cravings are almost gone for alcohol, sweets and chocolate! Thank goodness!

5. Have you noticed any change in your weight?
I lost a few pounds that I wanted to lose!

6. Did your sleep change?
A few times I needed less sleep, and get up less in the night.

7. Did your elimination change?
I have been going to the bathroom more times each day. For 1½ weeks I have had very loose bowels. Some diarrhea in the mornings.

8. Did your energy change?
More energy! I wake up and jog at 6 a.m. before working at 7 a.m.

9. Did anybody comment on how you looked?
Someone thought I lost weight and looked fine. I inspired some others by my enthusiasm!

10. Did you have any symptoms of detox?
Spots like pimples or rash (not hives)

Flu symptoms, some nausea when I would think about taking vitamins, diarrhea almost every morning for 10 days or so, a few aches and pains in joints.

11. Did you have any negative experiences?

Nothing negative at all.

12. Would you like to continue drinking Green Smoothies?

Yes! And I want to be 100% raw too!

Thank you so much!

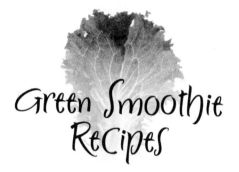

Green Smoothie Recipes

Sweet Green Smoothies

Raw Family Wild Banango

Blend well:
2 cups lambsquarters (plantain,
   chickweed or other weed)
1 banana
1 mango
2 cups water
Yields: 1 quart of smoothie

Blueberry Pudding

Blend well:
1 stalk of celery
2 cups fresh blueberries
1 banana
2 cups water
Yields: 1 quart of smoothie

Valya's Favorite
Blend well:
8 leaves of Romaine lettuce
5 cups watermelon
1 cup water
Yields: 1 quart of smoothie

Green Benevolence
Blend well:
6 to 8 leaves of Romaine lettuce
1 cup of red grapes
1 medium orange
1 banana
2 cups water
Yields: 1 quart of smoothie

Sweet and Sour
Blend well:
6 to 8 leaves of red leaf
4 apricots
1 banana
1/4 cup blueberries
2 cups water
Yields: 1 quart of smoothie

Freshness
Blend well:
6 to 8 leaves of Romaine lettuce
1/2 medium honeydew
2 cups water
Yields: 1 quart of smoothie

Aloe Live

Blend well:
1 cup apple juice
1 banana
1 mango
1 small piece of aloe
5 leaves of kale
2 cups water
Yields: 1 quart of smoothie

Mango–Parsley Pudding

Blend well:
2 large mangos (peeled)
1 bunch parsley
2 cups water
Yields: 1 quart of thick smoothie

Summer Delight

Blend well:
6 peaches (without seed)
2 handfuls of spinach leaves
2 cups water
Yields: 1 quart of smoothie

Weeds for Kids

Blend well:
4 mangos (peeled)
1 handful of lambsquarters (or other weed,
   like stinging nettles, purslane, etc)
2 cups water
Yields: 1 quart of sweet thick (like
   pudding) smoothie

Strawberry Field

Blend well:
1 cup strawberries
2 bananas
1/2 bunch romaine
2 cups water
Yields: 1 quart of smoothie

Chia Seed Green Pudding

Soak 1 Tbsp chia seeds for 1 hour
   in 1 cup of water.
In one hour you will have
   1 cup of chia jell.

Blend well:
1 cup of chia jell (1 Tbsp chia seeds,
   soaked for 1 hour in 1 cup of water)
1 Tbsp chia seeds (soaked for 1 hour
   in 1 cup of water)
4 apples (sweet and juicy kind, peeled)
1/2 lemon (juiced)
4–5 leaves of kale
1 sprig mint (optional)
2 cups water
Yields: 1 1/2 quart of thick smoothie

Kiwi Enjoyment

Blend well:
4 very ripe kiwis (green or golden)
1 ripe banana
3 stalks of celery
2 cups water
Yields: 1 quart of smoothie.

Igor's Favorite

Blend well:
1/2 bunch spinach
4 apples (peeled)
1/2 whole lime with peel
1 banana
2 cups water
Yields: 1 quart of smoothie

Minty Thrill

Blend well:
4 ripe pears
4–5 leaves of kale
1/2 bunch of mint
2 cups water
Yields: 1 quart of smoothie

10 Fingers

Blend well:
10 finger-bananas
2 handfuls of spinach leaves
2 cups water
Yields: 1 quart of smoothie

Raspberry Dream

Blend well:
2 bosc pears
1 handful of raspberries
4–5 leaves of kale
2 cups water
Yields: 1 quart of smoothie

Savory Green Smoothies

Victoria's Favorite

Blend well:
6 leaves of red leaf lettuce
1/4 bunch of fresh basil
1/2 lime (juiced)
1/2 red onion
2 celery sticks
1/4 avocado
2 cups water
Yields: 1 quart of smoothie

Sergei's Favorite

Blend well:
5 kale leaves (green)
1/2 bunch of fresh dill
1/2 lime (juiced)
3 cloves garlic
1/4 cup sun dried tomatoes
2 cups water
Yields: 1 quart of smoothie

Orion's Lemon Jalapeno Fresca

Blend well:
1/2 lemon (juice)
4 Roma tomatoes
2/3 bunch kale
1/2-inch jalapeno pepper
1 small clove garlic
2 cups water
Yields: 1 quart of smoothie

Shakti's Green Thai

Blend well:
2½ cups spinach
½ bunch cilantro
1 clove garlic
½ red bell pepper
½ lime (juiced)
1 tsp stevia (1 green leaf)
3 roma tomatoes
2 cups water
Yields: 1 quart of smoothie

Green Delicious

The whole point in making green smoothies is to consume more greens, especially without salt. However we included salt in this extraordinarily tasty recipe. We found it useful for treating those of our friends who eat a mainstream diet.

Blend well:
5 leaves of kale (purple)
¼ avocado
3 cloves garlic
juice of ½ lime
2 cups water
½ tsp. Salt
2 Roma tomatoes
Yields: 1 quart of smoothie

Nutritiously Bitter

Blend well:
5 leaves of kale (green or purple)
1/4 avocado
3 cloves garlic
1/4 cup lime juice
2 cups water
1 bell pepper
2 celery sticks
1/2 bunch of Italian parsley
2 cups water
Yields: 1 quart of smoothie

Important Tips

❧ Storage of Green Smoothies

While fresh is always best, green smoothies
will keep in cool temperatures for up to
three days, which can be handy at work
and while traveling.

❧ Rotation of Greens

I would like to emphasize the importance
of using a wide variety of greens. Try to get
a hold of as many different greens as you
can. If you continue to use the same greens,
you can expect to lose your desire for green
smoothies.

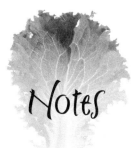

Notes

Chapter 3

1. Frequently Asked Questions. Chimpanzee and Human Communication Institute, 2004. Accessible at: http://www.cwu.edu/~cwuchci/faq.html

2. Derek E. Wildman, et al. "Implications of Natural Selection in Shaping 99.4% Nonsynonymous DNA Identity Between Humans and Chimpanzees: Enlarging Genus *Homo.*" Article in *Proceedings of the National Academy of Sciences,* May 19, 2003 (#2172) USA

3. Ibid.

4. James Q. Jacobs. "A Comparison of Some Similar Chimpanzee and Human Behaviors." *Paleoanthropology in the 1990's.* 2000. Accessible at: www.jqjacobs.net

5. Chimpanzees. World Wildlife Fund. Washington, DC. 2005. Accessible at: http://intothewild.tripod.com/chimpanzees.htm

6. Louis R. Sibal and Kurt J. Samson. "Nonhuman Primates: A Critical Role in Current Disease Research." *ILAR Journal* V42(2) 2001. Accessible at: http://dels.nas.edu/ilar/jour_online/42_2/nhprole.asp

7. Ibid.

8. Frequently Asked Questions. Chimpanzee and Human Communication Institute, 2004. Accessible at: http://www.cwu.edu/~cwuchci/faq.html

9. Nancy Lou Conklin-Brittain, Richard W. Wrangham, Catherine C. Smith, *Relating Chimpanzee Diets to Potential Australopithecus Diets,* Department of Anthropology, Harvard University, Cambridge, MA. 1998. Accessible at: www.cast.uark.edu/local/icaes/conferences/wburg/posters/nconklin/conklin.html

10. Goodall, Jane. *The Chimpanzees of Gombe*. Massachusetts: The Belknap Press of Harvard University Press. 1986.

11. Nancy Lou Conklin-Brittain, Richard W. Wrangham, Catherine C. Smith, *Relating Chimpanzee Diets to Potential Australopithecus Diets*, Department of Anthropology, Harvard University, Cambridge, MA. 1998. Accessible at: www.cast.uark.edu/local/icaes/conferences/wburg/posters/nconklin/conklin.html

Chapter 4

12. Price, Weston A., D.D.S. *Nutrition and Physical Degeneration*. California: The Price-Pottenger Nutrition Foundation, Inc. 2003. 6th Edition.

13. Ibid.

Chapter 5

14. U.S. Department of Agriculture, Agricultural Research Service. 2005. USDA National Nutrient Database for Standard Reference, Release 18. Accessible at: http://www.nal.usda.gov

Chapter 6

15. Shelton, Herbert M. *Dr. Shelton's Hygienic Review*. Pomeroy: Health Research, 1996

16. Dietary Reference Intakes for Males, aged 19–30. National Research Council, "Protein and Amino Acids," in *Recommended Dietary Allowances*, 10th edition (1989); USDA SR17

Chapter 7

17. Nancy Lou Conklin-Brittain, Richard W. Wrangham, Catherine C. Smith, *Relating Chimpanzee Diets to Potential Australopithecus Diets*, Department of Anthropology, Harvard University, Cambridge, MA. 1998.

18. Data from Average Adult Male, Age 19–31, Weight 170 lbs. Source: National Research Council, "Protein and Amino Acids," in *Recommended Dietary Allowances*, 10th edition (1989); USDA SR17

19. Walker WA, Isselbacher KJ. "Uptake and transport of macro-molecules by the intestine. Possible role in clinical disorders." *Gastroenterology*: 67:531–50, 1974

20. Ross, Julia, M.A. *The Diet Cure*. New York: Penguin Books. 1999.

21. U.S. Department of Agriculture, Agricultural Research Service. 2005. USDA National Nutrient Database for Standard Reference, Release 18

22. Campbell, T. Colin, Ph.D. *The China Study.* Texas: Benbella Books 2004.

Chapter 8

23. Jensen Bernard, D.C., Ph.D. *Tissue Cleansing Through Bowel Management,* Escondido, CA: Bernard Jensen Publishing, 1981

24. Chopra, Deepak. *Perfect Health: the Complete Mind Body Guide.* New York: Three Rivers Press, 2000

25. Nancy Lou Conklin-Brittain, Richard W. Wrangham, Catherine C. Smith, *Relating Chimpanzee Diets to Potential Australopithecus Diets,* Department of Anthropology, Harvard University, Cambridge, MA. 1998.

26. Mosséri, Albert. Le Jeûne, Meilleur. *Remède de la Nature.* France: Aquarius, 1993

27. American Heart Association. *Fiber.* Accessible at: www.americanheart.org.

28. Tooshi, Dr. Alan M., Ph.D. *Dr. Tooshi's High Fiber Diet.* Nebraska: iUniverse.com, Inc. 2001.

29. Winick, Myron, M.D. *The Fiber Prescription.* New York: Ballantine Books. 1992.

30. American Heart Association, 2004. Accessible at: www.americanheart.org.

Chapter 9

31. Jensen, Bernard, D.C., Ph.D. *The Healing Power of Chlorophyll.* Escondido, CA: Bernard Jensen Publishing, 1981

32. Cannon, Walter B. *The Wisdom of the Body.* New York: Peter Smith Pub Inc, 1932

Chapter 10

33. Walker WA, Isselbacher KJ. "Uptake and Transport of Macro-molecules By the Intestine. Possible Role in Clinical Disorders." *Gastroenterology* 1974; 67:531–50.

34. Minocha Anil M.D., Carrol David. *Natural Stomach Care: Treating and Preventing Digestive Disorders with the Best of Eastern and Western Healing Therapies.* New York: Penguin Group, 2003

35. Elson M. Haas M.D. *Staying Healthy With Nutrition.* California: Celestial Arts, 1992.

36. Nancy Lou Conklin-Brittain, Richard W. Wrangham, Catherine C. Smith, *Relating Chimpanzee Diets to Potential Australopithecus Diets,* Department of Anthropology, Harvard University, Cambridge, MA. 1998. Accessible at: www.cast.uark.edu/local/icaes/conferences/wburg/posters/nconklin/conklin.html

37. Stiteler L. Ac., O.M.D., N.M.D., D. *A Closer Look at Hypochlorhydria.* Stephen, Hom. California: The Institute of Bioterrain sciences, 2003. Accessible at: http://www.csupomona.edu/%7Esteven/articles/hypochlorhydria-Stiteler.html

38. Baroody, Dr. Theodore A., Jr. *Alkalize or Die.* North Carolina: Eclectic Press. 1991.

39. Ibid.

Chapter 12

40. The Associated Press. "Cancer now the top killer of Americans" *USA Today,* January 20, 2005

41. Dr. Otto Warburg. K. Triltsch. *The Prime Cause and Prevention of Cancer.* 2d. rev. edition (1969) 16 pages. Lecture delivered to Nobel Laureates on June 30, 1966 at Lindau, Lake Constance, Germany. English Edition by Dean Burk National Cancer Institute, Bethesda, Maryland, USA. Accessible at: http://www.mmfnd.org/NL/ONN/WS/ozon005.html

42. Ibid.

43. Baroody, Dr. Theodore A., Jr. *Alkalize or Die.* North Carolina: Eclectic Press. 1991.

Chapter 13

44. Tompkins, Peter and Bird, Christopher. *The Secret Life of Plants.* New York: Harper & Row, Publishers. 1989. First Perennial Library Edition.

45. Tompkins, Peter and Bird, Christopher. *Secrets of the Soil.* Anchorage, Alaska: Earthpulse Press Inc. 2002. Third Printing.

46. Tompkins, Peter and Bird, Christopher. *The Secret Life of Plants.* New York: Harper & Row, Publishers. 1989. First Perennial Library Edition.

47. Vyapaka Dasa, organic farm inspector. *It Ain't Just Dirt!* Canada, 2005. Accessible at: http://www.hkrl.com/soils.html

48. Farr, Gary, Dr. *Comparing Organic Versus Commercially Grown Foods,* Rutgers University Study, New Brunswick, NJ, 2002.

49. Tompkins, Peter and Bird, Christopher. *Secrets of the Soil.* Anchorage, Alaska: Earthpulse Press Inc. 2002. Third Printing.

50. Blume David. "Food and Permaculture." Article at: http://www.permaculture.com/permaculture/About_Permaculture/ food.shtml

51. Ibid.

52. Kervran, Louis. *Biological Transmutations.* London: Crosby Lockwood, 1972.

53. Tompkins, Peter and Christopher Bird. *The Secret Life of Plants.* New York: Harper & Row, Publishers. 1989. First Perennial Library Edition.

54. Ibid.

55. Korolkov, P. A. *Spontaneous Metamorphism of Minerals and Rocks.* Moscow: Nauka, 1972.

Chapter 14

56. Warburg, Otto. "The Oxygen-Transferring Ferment of Respiration." Nobel Lecture, 1931. From *Nobel Lectures, Physiology or Medicine 1922–1941,* Amsterdam: Elsevier Publishing Company, 1965

57. *Chlorophyllin Reduces Aflatoxin Indicators Among People At High Risk For Liver Cancer.* Johns Hopkins University Bloomberg School of Public Health. Baltimore, MD. Proceedings of the National Academy of Sciences. November 27, 2001.

58. Chernomorsky, S. et al. "Effect of Dietary Chlorophyll Derivatives on Mutagenesis and Tumor Cell Growth." *Teratogenesis, Carcinogenesis, and Mutagenesis,* 79:313–322, 1999.

59. Vlad M. et al. *Effect of Cuprofilin on Experimental Atherosclerosis.* Romania: Institute of Public Health and Medical Research, University of Medicine and Pharmacy, Cluj-Napoca, 1995

Chapter 15

60. Soloukhin, Vladimir. Razryv Trava. In Russian. Moscow: Molodaya Gvardia, 2001.

61. Goodall, Jane. *The Chimpanzees of Gombe*. Massachusetts: The Belknap Press of Harvard University Press. 1986.

62. Baker Elizabeth. *Unbelievably Easy Sprouting!* Washington: Poulsbo, 2000.

Chapter 16

63. Ruimerman, Ronald. *Modeling and remodeling in bone tissue*. Eindohoven. University Press Facilities. 2005.

64. Sartin, Daniel. "Osteoporosis: Why Prevention is the Best Cure." *Touching Lives: Action Medical Research*. Winter 2003/4.

65. Nishimura Ichiro. *Getting to the Roots of the Jaw Bone*. Dentistry Harvard, 1995, May12.

66. Price, Weston A., D.D.S. *Nutrition and Physical Degeneration*. California: The Price-Pottenger Nutrition Foundation, Inc. 2003. 6th Edition.

Chapter 17

67. Van Orden, Dr. Flora. *Conversations with Dr. Flora*. Florida: TheRawDiet.com. 2005.

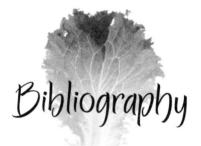

Bibliography

Albi, Johnna and Walthers, Catherine. *Greens Glorious Greens!* New York: St. Martin's Press. 1996.

Appleton, Nancy. *Rethinking Pasteur's Germ Theory.* California: North Atlantic Books. 2002.

Baker, Elizabeth. *Unbelievably Easy Sprouting!* Washington: Elizabeth Baker. 2000.

Baroody, Dr. Theodore A., Jr. *Alkalize or Die.* North Carolina: Eclectic Press. 1991.

Brown, Ellen Hodgson, J.D. and Hansen, Richard T., D.M.D., FACAD. *The Key to Ultimate Health.* California: Advanced Health Research Publishing. 2000. 2nd Edition.

Campbell, T. Colin, Ph.D. *The China Study.* Texas: Benbella Books 2004.

Cooper, Dr. Kenneth H. *Advanced Nutritional Therapies.* Tennessee: Thomas Nelson, Inc. 1996.

Cutrell, Doug and Wigmore, Ann. *Living Foods Manual.* New Mexico.

Feldt, Linda Diane. *Spinach and Beyond.* Michigan: Moon Field Press. 2003.

Fouts, Roger. *Next of Kin.* New York: HarperCollins Publishing. 2003 Reprint.

Fuhrman, Joel, M.D. *Eat to Live*. New York: Little, Brown and Company. 2003.

Gebhardt, Susan E. and Thomas, Robin G. *Nutritive Value of Foods*. Washington, D.C.: Superintendent of Documents U.S. Government Printing Office. 2002. Revised.

Goodall, Jane. *Reason For Hope*. New York: Warner Books, Inc. 1999.

———. *The Chimpanzees of Gombe*. Massachusetts: The Belknap Press of Harvard University Press. 1986.

———. *Through a Window*. Boston: Houghton Mifflin Company. 1990.

Harris, Ben Charles. *Eat the Weeds*. Connecticut: Keats Publishing, Inc. 1973.

Jensen, Bernard, DC, Ph.D. *Come Alive!* California: Bernard Jensen, 1997.

———. *Tissue Cleansing Through Bowel Management*. Escondido, CA: Bernard Jensen Publishing, 1981

Kliment, Felicia Drury, *The Acid Alkaline Balance Diet*. New York: Contemporary Books, 2002.

Krishnamurti. *Think on These Things*. New York: Harper & Row Publishers. 1964.

Ladygina-Kohts, N.N. *Infant Chimpanzee and Human Child*. New York: Oxford University Press, Inc. 2002.

Ley, Beth M. Ph.D. *Flax! Fabulous Flax!* Minnesota: BL Publications. 2003.

Mindell, Earl, R.Ph., Ph.D. *Food as Medicine*. New York: Simon & Schuster. 1994.

Peterson, Lee Allen. *Edible Wild Plants*. New York: Houghton Mifflin Company. 1977.

Price, Weston A., D.D.S. *Nutrition and Physical Degeneration*. California: The Price-Pottenger Nutrition Foundation, Inc. 2003. 6th Edition.

Ragnar, Peter. *How long do you choose to live?* Tennessee: Roaring Lion Publishing. 2001.

Ross, Julia, M.A. *The Diet Cure*. New York: Penguin Books. 1999.

Ruimerman, Ronald. *Modeling and remodeling in bone tissue*. Eindohoven: University Press Facilities. 2005.

Seibold, Ronald L. M.S. *Cereal Grass.* Kansas: Pines International, Inc.2003.

Shahani, Khem, Ph.D. *Cultivate Health from Within.* Connecticut: Vital Health Publishing, 2005.

Stanway, Dr. Andrew. *The High-Fiber Diet Book.* New York: Exeter Books. 1976.

Tompkins, Peter and Bird, Christopher. *Secrets of the Soil.* Anchorage, Alaska: Earthpulse Press Inc. 2002. Third Printing.

————. *The Secret Life of Plants.* New York: Harper & Row, Publishers. 1989. First Perennial Library Edition.

Tooshi, Dr. Alan M., Ph.D. *Dr. Tooshi's High Fiber Diet.* Nebraska: iUniverse.com, Inc. 2001.

Van Orden, Dr. Flora. *Conversations with Dr. Flora.* TheRawDiet.com. 2005.

Wigmore, Dr. Ann and Earp-Thomas, Dr. G.H. *Organic Soil.* Massachusetts: Rising Sun Publications. 1978.

Wigmore, Ann. *Overcoming Aids.* New York: Copen Press. 1987.

————. *Rebuild Your Health.* Puerto Rico: Quality Printers. 1991.

————. *You Are The Light Of The World.* Massachusetts: Ann Wigmore. 1990.

Wigmore, Ann and Pattinson, Lee. *The Blending Book.* New York: Avery Publishing Group. 1997.

Winick, Myron, M.D. *The Fiber Prescription.* New York: Ballantine Books. 1992.

Young, Robert O. and Shelly Redford. *The pH Miracle.* New York: Warner Books, Inc. 2002.

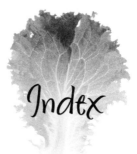

Index

Order Form

For books by
Raw Family Publishing

Online orders: **www.RawFamily.com**

E-mail: **Victoria@rawfamily.com**

Postal orders:
Raw Family Publishing, P.O. Box 172, Ashland, OR 97520

Phone: (541) 488-8865

Please send [   ] copies of *Green For Life* @ $14.95

Please send [   ] copies of *12 Steps to Raw Food* @ $16.95 (new!)

Please send [   ] copies of *Raw Family* @ $9.95

Please send [   ] copies of *Eating Without Heating* @ $11.95

Please send [   ] copies of DVD *Greens Can Save Your Life* –
Bestseller! (Three-hour lecture on 2 discs, nicely complements the
book) 2005 @ $24.95

Please send [   ] copies of DVD *Raw Gourmet Dishes Simplified*
(Victoria teaches how to prepare 14 basic raw dishes) 2003 @ $19.95

Please send [   ] copies of audio CD *Spiritual Awakening with Raw
Foods* (Victoria shares her unique perspective on the connection
between spirituality and diet) 2004 @ $11.95

Shipping and handling: $3.50 for the first book or DVD and $1.00
for each additional

Payment: Check or money order   **Total $**_____

Name: _____

Address: _____

City: _____ State: _____ Zip: _____

Telephone: _____

E-mail address: _____

Wholesale discounts available on large quantities.